For This Child We Prayed:
Living with the Secret Shame of Infertility

Lena M. Fields-Arnold

*IN*fertility Press
Dayton, OH

For This Child We Prayed:
Living with the Secret Shame of Infertility

Copyright © 2006

Lena M. Fields-Arnold

All Rights Reserved.
No part of this book may be reproduced or transmitted in any form or by any means, electrical or mechanical, including photocopying and recording, or by any information storage or retrieval systems except as may be expressly permitted by the Copyright Act or in writing from the author/publisher.

ISBN: 978-0-9795613-0-6
Library of Congress Control Number: 2007930245

Published by *IN*fertility Press
Cover Photo & Layout by Val Ragland/www.JeffreyAllanPhotography.com
Cover Conversion & Layout Elaine Lanmon

*All Scripture quotations unless otherwise noted are taken from either The Authorized Kings James Version of the Bible or *The Word In Life*™ Study Bible: New Kings James Version Published by Thomas Nelson, Copyright 1993, 1996.

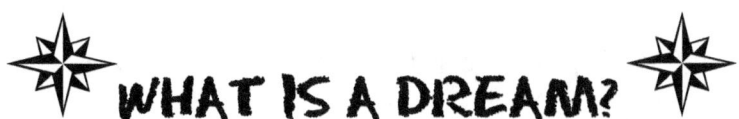
WHAT IS A DREAM?

"A dream is a personal love letter given to us by God.
He writes it on our heart that we may begin to wonder of His greatness
and of the potential that was placed in us before birth.

Like a love letter it is written expressly
to you from your loved one,
and holds a special meaning for you alone.
When shared with the world before its time,
it is not understood.
But when it's revealed by your
expression of hope and love and joy,
it is then and only then a dream that has come true."

Horace Arnold, Jr.

"For I considered all this in my heart,
so that I could declare it all: that the righteous and the wise
and their works are in the hand of God."
Ecclesiastes 9:1

Contents

Thoughts of Love Appreciation and Support 5

Foreword by Dr. Carolyn L. Gordon 6

Understanding Alma 7

1: Waiting on God: Journeys through Past Pain 10

2: Will Somebody Please Hand Me an Umbrella? 34

3: Year of Jubilee is the Year of Grief to Me 48

4: TKO: Trusting God When You're Gittin' Beat Down 66

5: When the Clouds Move-Faith Appears 73

6: Calling on God When Your Strength is Gone 124

7: Praising God in the Sunshine 147

8: Living Life without the Secret Shame 177

The Finish 192
Epilogue 193
About the Author 195
Resources 196
Notes and Helpful Websites 197

Thoughts of Love, Appreciation, and Support

Horace Arnold-My Husband
Your unconditional love and support has been my strength. When I wanted to throw in the towel you wouldn't let me. You truly are my better half.
I love you.

Selener Jones Fields- My Mother
The strongest woman I ever knew.
Thanks for teaching me how to be a mother.

Chrystal Fields-Elebesunu & Mary Arnold
Thanks for mothering me.

Marion Witcher, Janet Corney, Tina Spears, Kim Winters, Angie Whitfield, Tracee Arnold, Carolyn Gordon, Craig & Kimya, friends & family.
Thanks for the great friendship, advice and support-I love you.

Jimmy & Mark-My Brothers-and all my brothers and sisters-in-law.
It feels good to know that you always have my back!

Fellow Soldiers on the Infertility Battlefield
With God all things are possible.

Revival Center Ministries International
Goad International Ministries
Joshua Christian Ministries
I remember your example and prayers-thanks and God bless.

Dr. Keith Watson and Staff
Thanks for all you've done! You are a credit to your profession.

Kettering Reproductive Medicine
www.kmcnetwork.org/wcs/KRM.cfm
Drs. Bidwell, Burwinkle, and St. Pierre, Betheen, BSN, RN
The best doctors, nurses, and staff! Thanks for being dedicated and caring.

Penda L. Horton-James, InSCRIBEd Inspirations
Thanks for helping to deliver my dream! Your gifts will make room for you.

Foreword

By Rev. Dr. Carolyn L. Gordon, PhD.

Gifts from God do not always come in pleasant packages wrapped in beautiful silk paper with awe-inspiring bows. Sometimes the gift comes through much pain, agony and questioning. Such is the case with Lena's struggle through infertility. In our society, being single and childless is painful, yet acceptable. To have a husband and be childless because your body has turned on you is often perceived to be an act of punishment from God. The unspoken condemnation is, that *"somebody did something wrong, somewhere."* Even Biblically, God is portrayed as one who rewards women with children who are obedient to him. Such was the case with the two Hebrew midwives who were commanded by Pharaoh to kill all Hebrew male babies at birth. Shiphrah and Puah refused to obey the monarch and very creatively conjured up a way of explaining their insubordination. In return for their faithfulness, the Old Testament scriptures suggest that God rewarded them with children.

"So God was kind to the midwives and the people increased and became even more numerous. And because the midwives feared God, he gave them families of their own." Exodus 1:20-21.

Thus, the assumption is that if a woman or man cannot have children; it must not only be God's will, but true evidence of God's wrath in action. In this book, Lena dispels this horrendous misconception through personal insight, reflection and God given synergy. In her struggle to have children, she invites us to journey with her. It is a tremendous journey, which takes us through the heartache of a crying, barren womb to sitting with Hannah in the scriptures as she bargains with God for a child…to the man at the pool of Bethesda who experienced the miracle of Christ's healing…to her own personal thoughts as she writes to her future children like Celie wrote to Nettie in Alice Walker's book *"The Color Purple."* It is a journey of discovering the true will of God for her life while recognizing the fact that she was not alone in her travails. The journey begins anew with the divine revelation that God can work in more than one way: Just because she— Lena was barren, it did not mean that it was God's will for her to be chronically and eternally childless. God always has a way, a will and a plan; it is simply ours to trust Him and the process.

Understanding Alma

I was 12 years old in 1978 when Louise Brown, the first "test tube baby" was born. I clearly remember being fascinated about a baby being conceived in a tube. Already just beginning to understand the concept of reproduction, this new method was too much for me to fathom. As I grew into a young adult and learned more and more about the myriad forms of *alternative conception* I began to philosophize that these forms were somehow abnormal.

Now as a young adult, who'd grown up on Christian theology I had a tendency to see things only in black and white. "There is only one way to conceive," I thought, and though inherently I wasn't opposed to In-Vitro fertilization I just theorized that it wasn't for me. The concepts of sperm samples, sperm and egg donation, and surrogacy even more muddled the waters of my growing judgments. And when you mixed all that with court battles and ethics I simply chalked it all up as one big mess and that women with sense ought to just leave it all alone and accept whatever fate God dealt them.

But then I was young, did not want children, and was naïve to the fact that I might someday become one of the women I had previously scorned in my judgments.

So it would seem that having babies is the most natural thing in the world, but for the couples in this country experiencing infertility issues, (of which I was now one) becoming and staying pregnant can be extremely overwhelming and emotionally taxing, not to mention the financial burden placed on already beleaguered couples.

Most women who endure the trial of infertility feel alone, as if there is no one with whom we can share our secret grief, for we mourn each month for the loss of the hope of life, of a future, of an expected end. We go through each stage of grief alone. We spend years denying we have a problem, and then when we finally admit it many of us are angry.

How many times have I shaken my fist at God and yelled, "Why me?" Over and again I lashed out at my husband, "Why don't you seem to be as upset about this as I am?"

How many doctors have I blamed, "Why didn't you find out what was wrong with me?" And how many times have I been angry with myself questioning, "Why don't you work right?"

I felt powerless, and this powerlessness led to depression and grief. Month after month I mourned over my loss, or rather my lack of loss. I wanted to end it all, all the suffering, all the misery, all the heartache…

Traditionally, infertility has been referred to as the "woman's problem" totally ignoring the male contribution. Though the reality is that infertility affects males and females equally, it is usually the woman who feels the brunt of the pain, for it is the woman who is bound the motherhood mandate and feels the pressure to procreate.

Sandra Glahn in her book with Dr. William Cutrer, *When Empty Arms Become a Heavy Burden: Encouragement for Couples Facing Infertility,* discussed how little girls play with dolls and hear their mothers say, "'When you have a daughter…' They grow up assuming they will bear children…Males receive a different cultural message, that if you have a family fine, if you have a job better…women grow up thinking that motherhood is the central role in their lives… and it stands to reason that the effects of infertility identity would be more severe on them."

As an African American Christian couple we faced a double whammy, seeing that in the black Christian community families are more important than careers and manhood is defined by the ability to procreate. So in essence, I was fighting a battle within a battle, within a battle.

And just what was it I was battling? I was fighting a mean disorder of the reproductive system that impairs the body's ability to conceive a baby or sustain a pregnancy; affecting males and females in equal numbers, and in a few cruel cases-both partners. In others there is no known cause, further adding to the heartache.

> *"There is no visible injury, no disease, no dear relative or friend to mourn, only a deep wound in my psyche, a hole where a child might have been. To many this seems like a peculiar overreaction. To me and us and to those like us it is neither. It is real. I had built a not uncommon fantasy, but a wish has no form, and everything seems to remind you of it. There are no rituals to guide your mourning, no headstone in a cemetery."*—
> Alma-From <u>When Empty Arms Become A Heavy Burden</u>

I am like Alma. I buried a child in my heart every month for more than ten years before I finally admitted that this was a problem beyond the scope of my reach. The grief was compounded by renewed hope each month and the reality that there was nothing I could do to "fix" myself. I was forced to find some way to cope with this ongoing process of grief. It was this "coping" that made life unbearable because I lived life in a fog of uncertainty. I couldn't plan my future because I was too focused on the now. Thoughts like, "I can't take this job," or "I can't start graduate school because I might get pregnant and have to quit," kept me stagnant. Thus, hope became my enemy as my spirit was worn down from the incessant battle.

My dream was dying, and with it a piece of me. So I began to write.

This journal is my weapon, the words are the stones, and the act of writing is my practice. Through them I will conquer this enemy of infertility and overcome the sadness, depression, despair. It is my most sincere desire that it will help you triumph over those enemies as well.

Lena

CHAPTER 1

Waiting on God: Journeys through Pain

"Wait on the Lord; be of good courage, and He shall strengthen your heart: Wait I say, on the Lord."
Psalms 27:14

Elizabeth

I see the children playing
And I wish one could be mine
I know if I just trust God
He'll give me one in time
I hear the children laughing
And I know how Sarah felt
I thought of all these things
As I bowed to God and knelt
Then I heard His tender voice
whisper gently in my ear,

"I know the pain inside your heart
And when you pray I hear
I know of the tears of sadness
You cry to me each day
Long ago a teary eyed Rebekah
Cried out to me this way
I wiped away Rachel's tears
And comforted Hannah's crying at my breast
I dried their eyes and held them
As I promised them they'd be blessed
Their house was not left barren
And neither will yours be my dear
Just keep on trusting in me,
The Living God, because I hear
I hear you when you laugh my child
I hear you when you cry
I delivered you to your mom at birth
I'll receive you when you die
I am the Almighty
The Living God above
I am the one who shelters you
And shows you greater love
I keep you and protect you
Holding you so tenderly
Everywhere you are,
You are a part of me
Don't ever get so discouraged
To feel that I'm not near
Just keep on trusting in me
The Living God
Because I HEAR"

"Trust in the Lord, and do good; so shall you dwell in the land and truly you shall be fed. Delight yourself also in the Lord and he shall give you the desires of your heart. Commit your way unto the Lord; trust also in Him and He will bring it to pass..."
Psalm 37: 3-7

September 13, 1995

Dear God:

How the hell much longer must I wait!!!

Yesterday I bought two picture frames as a testament of my faith. One for my niece Ivory who was born three months premature, that she will come home and one for the child I have been waiting on for *five years now!*

I caught your daddy winding the frame that plays the tune, *"This Old Man..."* How much longer must he wait Lord?

I'm sorry Father, I know I don't sound very Christian right now, but I can't help the way I feel.

Mom told me that when I was born I came out with my fist balled up and looked like I was ready to fight. She said that when I gave my life to You I'd understand why You made me a fighter and that I would use this trait to win souls for You. Well guess what, I don't feel like fighting, and I sure as hell don't feel like winning any damned souls!

Then from somewhere I hear, "You've got three choices: run, stand there and get pummeled, or do your best to fight and win."

Well God– I'm trying, but give me the strength, 'cause I sure don't have my own.

Love Lena

"It is better to trust in the Lord than to put confidence in man."
Psalm 118:8

October 17, 1995

Dear Children:

And that's how it started. A loving God, who gave me the strength to carry on, through an inborn trait, led me to this place of writing to you.

I often fantasize about everything, that's why it hurts so much waiting for you to arrive. It hurts to watch the months turn into years. It hurts to learn to trust God, but some of the greatest lessons in life are learned through pain and trials. Through these trials, God is fashioning me into a warrior — the kind I was born to be.

As God uses affliction to help us grow we wait. We don't always rest while we are waiting, nor are we always patient; those are things that must be learned. We pray and ask for God's help to rest and wait *patiently*. Then we develop trust and as learn to trust we feel a love for God that transcends even our miniscule understanding.

But it's still tough, I won't lie to you. Let me tell you from time to time someone will "*prophesy*" that you are coming soon. Sometimes I think people make things "*come from God*" but it's really just well meaning people wanting to make you feel better. Their words sound good to our ears so we think, "Yeah, that must be God," but it isn't. It hurts when someone says things like this and it doesn't happen. "Why did you let that person come to me?" I ask. "Why would you allow me to be hurt in this manner? And what does *soon* mean anyway?"

For example in August we went to visit a relative in Washington D.C. She told me, "God is telling me you are going to be pregnant soon." So when my period came I was very *dis*couraged. I had to force myself not to cry. Earlier I'd done a Bible study on trusting, which encouraged me despite my bruised heart.

Did God really speak to my cousin, or did she say what she thought I wanted to hear? It didn't help that I'd had this dream two weeks before. In it I was sad because I'd started my cycle. Then, I heard a voice saying to me, *"Don't be discouraged by what you see."*

Was the voice God's or my own subconscious? Often it's difficult to tell. Sometimes you just know because His voice is so clear and audible and you feel the Holy Spirit's urging. Other times it's a voice that comes from within. That's when it gets confusing because sometimes it sounds like you and so you wonder, "Is this really God, or am I hearing what I want to hear because I want it so badly?"

I don't want to be one of those people so I prepare myself for the agony, just in case. I thank God for the TODAY peace. I know from past experience the dark days will return. For today I will not lose my faith in God. Oh, yes, there are moments when you want to give up praying, thinking, "God you don't hear me anyway, so what's the point? Why should I even bother?"

> *"Trust in the Lord with all thy heart and do not lean unto your own understanding; but in all your ways acknowledge Him and He shall direct your paths."*
> **Proverbs 3:5, 6**

But you know what; maybe, just maybe harvest time is about to occur regarding our prayers. The Bible says in Ecclesiastes that to everything there is a season: *seedtime* (prayers) and *harvest* (answers.) After five years could it be that our harvest time is coming?

I trust You Lord but it ain't always easy. Then I hear a voice say, "Childlike faith means believing that there is nothing God cannot do, and trusting that He is willing to do it."

But what does all that mean? **Faith** (Hebrews 11 and 12:1-4)
It's acting upon what you believe: *I write to you — I believe you will be.*

It is a confident assurance that something we want is going to happen: *And we have begun to act upon that confidence by speaking of you as if you were already here.*

Faith is the certainty that what we hope for is waiting for us, even though we can't see it (physically) ahead: *I am certain God already knows you and when He plans to send you to us.*

Finally, it is being sure of things we hope for, knowing that "something" is real even though we cannot see, feel, or taste it: *You are real because I write in this journal, even though I can't yet see, feel, or hear you.*

Shortly after we married we turned our thoughts to having children. In my confused state of mind I thought having a child would be a magical Panacea that would make our marriage perfect. I was trying to use a child to do what only God could do: I thought that having a baby together would be a sign that I'd truly heard God about marrying your father.

I had plenty of reasons to justify my desire, but they were all carefully crafted lies. Deep down inside I didn't want the responsibilities that came with being a parent. So when the first year of our marriage passed and there was no child it really didn't bother either of us all that much.

> *"Lord, You have heard the desire of the humble; You will prepare their heart, You will cause Your ear to hear..."*
> **Psalm 10:17**

Now my prayers are different and I don't feel lucky.

"Father," I now pray in my most humble voice. "*In my innocence I have trusted you, and I have done well. I acknowledge that I don't understand why I must go through this and that I can't fix it. I ask you to heal us and to make us solid as only you can do. Help us to trust in you, now Lord, do your part and direct our path.*" (*That's what I pray when I'm feeling spiritual.*)

Love Mommy

"Is anything too hard for the Lord?"
Genesis 18:14 a

October 18th, 1995

Dear Children:

The last few months of 1991 and the first few months of 1992 were among the nastiest. What made the struggle worse was not having anyone to talk to about my problem. Talking to other people makes you feel like something is wrong with you. I wonder if they somehow think I am inadequate or if men sizing up my husband up as less than a man?

You don't want anyone to know what you're going through, because as soon as they know, accusations fly. I guess they think because we have been married five years and don't have children they somehow have the right to talk.
"What kind of underwear is Horace wearing?" Mark once asked.
"I am not discussing this with my little brother. I think to myself," but I answer anyway.
"He wears both boxers and briefs if you really must know."
"I'm just saying you know they say boxers are better."
"Don't worry; we've covered that base already."
"His pants aren't too tight are they?"
"What do you think?"
He laughed, "Have you guys thought about adopting?"
"Not again," I groaned.
"What did you say?"
"Nothing."
"Well, I wouldn't worry about it. With all of the things you guys have been doing for kids, I know God's going to give you some, one day. You guys are too great of a couple not to have kids." Ya, ya, ya!

After two years of interrogations like this I decided to see an infertility specialist. That's when I had my encounter with the doctor from Hell.

My friend Kimee recommended a doctor who was supposed to be "one of the best in Dayton." I don't know why I listened to her.

Right before the appointment I was having one of my world-famous pity parties with God invited as the guest of *dis*honor. I was in tears sniffing and sobbing, "God why me? Blah, blah, blah…"

Nevertheless I went full of hope and expectation, and instead what I got was a nightmare! Even while in the waiting room I felt as if I should leave. But, by then it was too late, they were calling my name. Mom and I walked into the office, paid the fee and went into the doctor's examination room to wait.

"I wonder why you aren't getting pregnant." Mom asked aloud, allowing her thoughts to be expressed as we looked around the room.

"According to this chart on the wall it could be a lot of things."

I said, walking over to it to get a closer look. "I could have blocked tubes, but I don't think so because that HSG test showed that they were clear. They could be infected though."

"I wonder what could infect your tubes."

"I don't know, but it also says that my vaginal fluids could be killing the sperm. Who would ever think their vagina would kill their husband's sperm?"

"That's something."

"His sperm could be bad, but I don't think so. I think I'm the problem."

"Why do you think it's you?" I tried to evade the question not wanting to answer it and examined the fetal growth charts, imagining one inside me. I really didn't think it was the right time to explain to her that I'd never used protection with my first fiancé, who now has kids.

"Why do you think it's you?" She asked again.

"Hi there, I'm Ruby." The nurse burst in at just the right moment. She smiled, "So, why are you here?" I explained.

"I assure you that Dr. Massicre is one of the most caring men I know. He will work with you and this will be one of the most wonderful doctor/patient relationships in the world!" She beamed.

"Why are you still dressed?" He burst in as she was still speaking.

"I wanted to talk to you first to be sure there is something you can do before I go through all this again."

"Well all right then." We made small talk for a few minutes, and he asked, "So what can I do for you?"

I proceeded to tell him my situation and reiterate to him the past history with doctors concerning this problem. Initially he seemed genuinely concerned. I told him the previous tests I had taken and asked if he could run all tests on me to find out if I was the problem.

"What?" He questioned. "You know it'll be cheaper to get your husband tested first to make sure he is not the problem before you spend a lot of money testing you?"

"Money isn't really a problem and I'm aware that there will be an expense to having me tested first, but I'm more comfortable going this route." He paused and gave me a strange look.

"Well what are your reasons for wanting to do it this way?"

I hesitated; embarrassed to admit the truth, that I was not a virgin when my husband and I met. I didn't want to acknowledge that I'd had sex with two other guys and had not gotten pregnant, though I'd never used birth control. I managed to get it out and quickly.

"Quite honestly, my husband and I have discussed it and with the way sperm samples are obtained we do not feel comfortable with him taking the test at this time." I didn't say we wouldn't do it, but we needed time to get to that place.

"This is the '90's and it's time people like you stopped buying into silly superstitions with regard to a medical test that could possibly save you a considerable amount of time and money."

"Look, I told you before that money isn't an issue. Now your nurse told me that you would be willing to work with me on my terms."

"Yes, but I don't understand why you're uncomfortable taking this test."

"I explained that already. Now will you help me determine whether or not something is wrong with me?"

"You're being silly and superstitious."

"I do not appreciate the way you are talking to me. You are starting to tick me off." I tried to keep calm, and mom tried to intervene before I totally lost it.

"No one can make you angry only you can make you angry." He spoke patronizingly.

"Don't talk to me as if I am some freshman college student and try to put this back on me." I say through clenched teeth.

"I came to you for help and you have done nothing but treat me like crap since I've been here. I won't take that from you or anyone else."

"Why? What have I done?" He asked innocently.

"You mock my religious beliefs and then accuse me of being silly and superstitious. You talk to me as if I am some stupid schoolgirl…"

"OK, OK let's try to start over." He interrupted. "What can I do for you?"

"What?"

"What can I do for you now? You don't want that test. What can I do for you?"

"Really, there is nothing you can do for me."

"No, really, what can I do for you?"

"The only thing you can do is give me my money back!"

"I'm trying to help you. You'll be back. Where are you going to go if I don't help you?"

"I don't want your help now. Why would I want you to help me, let alone deliver my child?"

"I don't understand. I was having a good day until I came in here. You're really messing up my day."

"No one can make you have a bad day. You are responsible for your own attitude. Isn't that what you're Psychology 101 book tells you?" Touché! I scored! I could tell by the look on his face!

This ordeal was horrible, and in spite of my successful barb, I was totally on edge. I had come to the professional for help. I was seeking understanding and compassion from a man who was supposed to have it and I didn't receive it. I wanted to die. Worse yet, I wanted to hurt him!

My energy was spent, but I could not let him see that. I had to make him think I didn't need him. How dare he talk to me this way? He's not God! Who does he think he is anyway?

"So you want your money back?" He said smiling a stupid grin.

"No problem, I don't need it." I got mad all over again. "But first, apologize for making me have a bad day."

"*Don't you dare!*" Mom mouths when she sees that I'm about to bash him with my purse.

"What!" I couldn't believe it, he wanted to humble me! This man knew I wasn't rich and $100 may not have been much to him, but it meant a lot to me. Ohh I was burning!

"You want me to apologize to you?" I held my purse tightly, "Well screw you." Deciding I'll repent later for anything I say.

"Yes, then I'll give your money back."

"I will kick your…"

"Marie!" Mom stopped me.

"Okay," I said to mom, then turned to him. "I'm sorry for ruining your ***stupid day,*** you insensitive idiot!"

"I'm sorry I couldn't help you."

"Whatever!" I said as we walked towards the office.

"I don't know what's wrong with her." He said to his secretary before telling her to give back my check. "She doesn't want my help." I was too angry to even reply.

Ruby saw the anger and hurt in my face and asked with concern.

"Are you going to be okay? Are you sure you don't want to try this?" She asked as she handed me my coat. I just played her off. "Well if you change your mind, if there's anything we can do for you just let me know."

"I doubt it," I said, trying to hold back the tears until I got out of the building. On the way out, I heard him talking to another patient as if I didn't even exist. As we walked out the door I thought I would burst.

I had so many thoughts, feelings, and emotions running through me that I couldn't even think straight. I couldn't do anything but sob uncontrollably. I was angry, hurt and full of questions. Why did this happen to me? This man was supposed to help me. This man was supposed to help me?

"The righteous cry and the Lord hears, and delivers them out of all their troubles."
Psalm 34:17

I struggled with the pain and mom tried her best to comfort me, but even she realized no words could have soothed my troubled soul.

She needed to pick up some things from the shopping center across the street, and I stayed in the van. While I waited for her, I looked up at the moon and stars that I've always loved and started crying.
I prayed, "Lord, you made the sky, moon, the stars, the world and everything in it. Surely it must be a small thing for you to give me a child. But if not I can accept that too, but You need to make it plain."

Looking up into that sky I understood the awesomeness of God.

He is everything I need Him to be and He is working out a perfect plan for our lives. How can we teach you to trust God if we haven't learned through experience?

When the disciples were in the storm on the Sea of Galilee they were terribly afraid and felt alone, but when Jesus came forth He said, "Be of good cheer: it is I; be not afraid." The storm was fulfilling the Word of God for their lives.

"Lord, thank You for the storm…, for it is the rain that makes flowers grow. Help us not to be concerned with the size of the problem, but rather let us see only the size of You. Give us direction and peace that by the world's standards we should not have."

As I looked up and prayed I was reminded to put on the whole armor of God and that the Lord is my rock, fortress, deliverer, and strength, and my high tower where I can find safety and protection in times of trouble.

Infertility often makes me feel like a loser, but, in Jesus I am victorious. Carolyn once asked me, "Marie if you are in the center of God's will, then where are you in a hurry to get to?" Good question. If I truly believe I am His, then I must also believe that I am in His will, even in the storm.

Love Mommy

*They that wait on the Lord shall renew their strength;
they shall mount up with wings like eagles.
They shall run and not get weary,
they shall walk and shall not faint."*
Isaiah 40:31

October 23, 1995

ARNOLD *"Strong as an Eagle"*

Dear Children:

I watched the TV show *"Coach"* tonight. He and his wife had been trying to have a child. They finally gave up and decided to adopt. It seems as if a lot of people have been doing shows or writing articles on this subject lately as if it's really increased within the last ten years. The last statistics I read said that about one in ten couples are infertile. That's pretty high!

It makes me wonder if *someone* is putting *something* in our food. As bad as my college fare was it wouldn't be hard for me to believe that something was put in that mess!

So anyway, I'm watching the show, and I'm feeling 'em, you know because people, who really mean well, have suggested we adopt too.

"Maybe God wants you to adopt." I recently replied to a friend who suggested that God wanted us to do so.

"We're not the ones experiencing problems with having kids. I'm just saying maybe God wants you be adoptive parents."

"So what you're saying is that only people who are experiencing infertility should adopt?"

"No, I'm just saying if you want kids you can always adopt them."

"I know you mean well, but adoption is not a cure for infertility. We'll adopt someday…"

"Well maybe God wants you to adopt first." She was undeterred.

Now I know she meant well, but I was not about to be deterred either. I paused for a second.

"If God wants us to adopt then He'd sure better hurry up and send ours because I'm not adopting any children until those by birth come first."

I'm not saying that's the right attitude, but that's how I felt at the moment.

"Okay then."

"If one more person tells me to adopt I am going to scream! If someone loses a child no one ever tells them to go adopt another one."

"Who else told you this?"

"My friend Kimee Jo," I love her dearly but she will get punched if she tells me one more time, 'Girl just go ahead and adopt and then you'll get pregnant, just like my friend Julie. There's something about adopting that helps you relax, like it makes your body want to be pregnant and then it cooperates. I'm telling you it happens all the time.'"

"Oh, I guess I can see why you are getting tired of hearing that."

"Well at least that's better than her telling me to have sex seven times a day then stand on my head afterwards."

"What! That is hilarious!" She laughed.

"Maybe to you, but not to me, she was serious."

On another occasion I heard.

"Well Lena, what if it's not God's will for you to have children? You know you have to be sure of that?" Alisa said.

Of course I didn't want to be out of God's will, but I'd received no indication from the Bible that it wasn't God's will. In fact, I'd drawn the conclusion, perhaps erroneously, that barrenness and infertility was most definitely not God's will. Now I'm not a theologian or anything but up until now I had no reason to think otherwise, though I might have to wait awhile.

"If it's not God's will for us to have children I would still serve Him, I mean I'd have to serve Him." I replied, "But I don't, I can't believe this is God's will. I am convinced we will have children." Shoot, she had four kids. What made her more worthy to receive children than me?

"Well at least you haven't been waiting twelve years like my parents. It all happens in God's time. You just have to be more patient.

Maybe that's what God is trying to teach you."

"More patient!" Oh Job I am truly feeling you my friend!

Sometimes you just don't want to hear words, not even from your well-meaning friends. I mean did she really think her words were encouraging me? C'mon, who wants to wait twelve years?

Initially, I wasn't even concerned, but into the second year of marriage and the second year of questions, I started to get worried.

When I started picking up weight and getting sick, I went to the gynecologist marking the beginning of the vicious *am I, am I not pregnant* cycle. I took a pregnancy test that came back negative. They ran some other tests and finally I was diagnosed.

"I have a urinary tract infection?" I questioned the doctor. "So I'm not pregnant? I mean, we've been married going on two years now and have never used birth control. Shouldn't I be pregnant by now?"

"It's not uncommon or abnormal, for it to take that long, I mean you're young and strong and there's no reason why you should not be getting pregnant. However I'll give you a prescription of Clomid to help ease your mind."

"What's that?"

"It's a fertility drug that will stimulate your ovaries to produce more eggs. If that doesn't work come back for another appointment."

The first prescription didn't work, so I went back the next month. I had gained more weight, and still had pains in my stomach area. A second pregnancy test came back negative, but an ultrasound revealed a small cyst on my left ovary.

We tried Clomid three times total before he put me on what he said was a *stronger hormone medication.** He said if that didn't work he would put me on even stronger fertility pills. I was getting a little concerned that he wasn't doing more to find out *why* I wasn't getting pregnant. Time was not on my side, I was getting older and I needed answers.

So I made an appointment with my previous Ob-Gyn for a

consultation and this time we both went.

"You'll have to come into the office and give us a sperm sample." He said to your daddy. "We have a room with some magazines if that will help."

"We'll have to think about that," He said.

"In the meantime we can go ahead and arrange to have your wife tested. I'll schedule a Hysterosalpinogram (HSG) to see if your tubes are blocked."

It was awful! They put you on this table and stick this long instrument between your legs and insert it into your vagina, up to your cervix, where it shoots some fluid into your tubes to see if it will go all the way through. If it doesn't go all the way through your tubes are blocked. You can watch it all on a monitor. My tubes were clear. Later on I felt so sick that I could not go to work. It was horrible!

This process of going to the doctor, only to be disappointed continued throughout the year. In between visits, I had to deal with physical and mental frustration and pain.

Usually, I would turn away from God instead of turning to Him, claiming I was too sick to pray. But the truth is my silence was my rebellion. I was too hurt by God to talk to Him. I would weep while having a soliloquy with Him.

"God I don't understand! I work with kids' everyday and give my heart to them, why can't I have one of my own?" I was hurting deeply and I didn't know what else to do.

> *"I once heard an old man say something that I have never forgotten. He said that when God tests you it is a good time for you to test Him by putting His promises to the proof. Claim from Him just as much as your trails have made necessary...recognize the trial as a challenge from God to claim a larger blessing than we have ever had."*— **A.B. Simpson**

I studied the Bible and found that God never left His people barren. No matter how long it took, God's people always conceived. I believed this was a promise to us and in my deepest moments of despair I clung to these promises.

"Lord, our current trials have made it necessary for me to claim from You wisdom and strength to endure. I don't pretend to know how You are going to make me a mother; I just know that You will. May I delight in You through the process and obtain a larger measure of Your grace."

Children, trust God no matter what you're going through.

Love Mommy

> *"In my distress I cried unto the Lord and He heard me."*
> ***Psalm 120:1***

November 10, 1995

Dear Children:

A friend suggested I should take a pregnancy test because I felt some crazy stuff going on inside my body. How could I explain to her that there's always something going on differently in my body! People say when you are pregnant you *just know, you feel unusual*. But how would I know? I always feel unusually sick!

Every time I have PMS, I'm convinced I'm pregnant. Any stomach virus I get can't wait to trick me and play emotional games with my head. I have even had psychosomatic symptoms. The slightest change in my physiological well-being will torment me, because I'm always looking for the slightest *"sign"* that will let me know.

During my lunch break I went to the store and purchased the test. All the while getting a little excited because maybe this time will be it! But just in case it isn't, I decide to begin seriously exercising. I figured if I can't get pregnant I might as well look good.

I went back work and put the test into the back of my mind. Later, after making sure your daddy was gone, I slipped into the bathroom to take it. There was no point in ruining his day if it was negative.

I was about to get started when he came back home looking for a hat. I threw the test into the cabinet above, just as he opened the bathroom door! But I left the box in the trashcan. I don't know how he missed it because it was sticking up from there in broad view. He left, but peeked in again just before I snatched the box from the trash and shoved it violently deep into one of the bathroom closets.

By now my bladder was really about to burst, but at last, finally I could take the test!

After a few minutes the results appeared. Remaining calm I picked up the test, and held onto it for a few minutes. Slowly I walked to the closet and pulled out the plastic bags and threw everything away. I feel nothing. I feel something. I feel empty. I want to cry, but I stop myself. I know I should run to God, but I don't. I don't know why. I'm not angry with Him. I just don't feel like talking. I just feel like doing nothing for a while. If it's wrong I can't help myself. I'm only running for a little while.

When I finally decided to turn to God I read in John 12:1-11, that many people came to see Lazarus in order to see with their own eyes the miracle Jesus had performed and many believed on Christ as a result.

But it seems that God isn't performing miracles like that any more. Well, I guess that's not really true. Maybe we don't see them because we expect God to do it our way, and when He doesn't we stop believing.

Do I really believe God will perform a Lazarus on me? Will He really raise up life in me? Do I really believe that Lazarus represents faith?

Bonita and I talked about it after dinner on Sunday while our husbands watched football.

"My neighbor has nine kids and wants more." She blurted out of nowhere.

"What, for real!" I exclaimed. Then, before I lost courage, "Speaking of kids, I've been thinking about buying an ovulation predictor test. What do you think about that?"

"It depends."

"Depends on what?" I asked even though I knew where she was going. Bonita understands exactly how I feel because two of her five pregnancies ended tragically and she still worried about subsequent ones.

"Well if you've already given it to God, and you totally trust Him then...I mean," She stuttered, "you might actually cause the blessing to be postponed if you try to *help* God, because that's what you're doing."

"Hmm," I sighed, wondering if God was really that petty. Is petty the right word to use?

"When we were trying to have kids we scheduled a bunch of tests to find out why we weren't conceiving. The day before the appointment my husband believed we shouldn't go and I reluctantly agreed. Shortly thereafter we discovered that I was already pregnant. I can see now that God was looking down from heaven at all our scrambling, wondering what we were doing and why we weren't waiting."

"Five years is a long time Bonita."

"Yes to us, but not to God. He can actually be getting ready to bless us and because we get ahead of Him He says, '*Well they haven't learned yet so we gotta take 'em through a little while longer.*'" She continued.

I wasn't sure how sound her arguments were, but I had no ammo with which to fight them. Sometimes I think we Christians have a tendency to say things that sound great but are not Biblically accurate. I mean think about it, do we really have the power to delay a blessing God intends to give us by grace? Maybe so, I don't know.

"It still sometimes seems like its unfair though doesn't it?" I asked.

"Yeah, but only God knows what we can handle and bear; maybe it's just not time. Who knows, your husband is going back to school and getting ready to quit his job?"

"I know. I know all that, but it still hurts."

"Yeah it does," she said.

"Especially when you see these teenage mothers getting pregnant and you think, "Lord, I don't understand, half these women don't even care about kids and I would be a good mother."

"I know," she laughed. "When my daughter died I thought I would never be able to go through anything like that, but God got us through it." She continued, "I remember when my best friend and I were the only ones at church who hadn't gotten pregnant yet. Then she got pregnant and I thought now I'm the only one."

Then I thought to myself, "Oh no! Her best friend's husband ate dinner with us and I'd stupidly said to him, "Isn't it time for your little boy to have a little brother or sister?" How could I of all people be so insensitive?

"Would you be willing to go through infertility treatments in order to conceive a child?" She interrupted my thoughts.

"Huh?" I said coming back to myself.

"Would be willing to go through infertility treatments?"

"I don't think I can handle that. I don't think I can handle all those shots."

"How bad do you want it?" She questioned.

"Very badly, but you just said God would not put more on us than we are able to bear." I laughed, "He knows I could never, EVER bear anything like that. I don't believe God would take me through all of that since He knows I could never, ever, ever bear it!"

"You'd be surprised what you can handle."

"I could NEVER handle that!"

"You never know how God's going to bring the blessing, but no matter how He chooses to do it, you need to keep on trusting Him and know that you are on the verge of a breakthrough."

Later that evening I prayed, *"Lord, may my confidence in You never waver. I'm beaten down emotionally and weak spiritually, but I know You have not forsaken me. You have begun this work and You will be faithful to complete it in us. Thank you Father, for You will perfect that which concerns me!"*

Love Mommy

*"In You, O' Lord, do I put my trust:
Let me never be put to confusion."*
Psalm 71:1

December 21, 1995

Dear Children:

"You know the Word says to call for the elders and let them pray and the prayer of faith will heal the sick." Kimee Jo said.

"I've heard that before, but Horace and I have studied that scripture. I've got to tell you, we're pretty convinced that it's talking about spiritual sickness, you know sin and stuff, not necessarily physical healing."

"What do you mean?"

"I mean, I read the chapters before and after that scripture. Everything is talking about living right, not sinning; being like Jesus and like Paul. One of the ways was calling for the elders and having them pray for you."

"I don't know about all that Lena."

"You went to college. You know how to study, read it yourself and you'll see what I'm talking about."

"Are you saying God doesn't heal?"

"No I'm not saying that. I'm just saying that's not really an accurate application of scripture to convince people that He does. I totally believe God heals; if I didn't, I don't think I could make it."

"Then what difference does it make if it's that scripture or another? If prayer will help why are you letting pride get in the way?

"It makes a difference if you're trying to use scripture to help someone. Yes, it's humbling to share such a deep personal problem as infertility—*and* sometimes I do feel ashamed because it's not an easy thing to ask for prayer about, but the main thing is I don't trust people to keep my secret. I don't want my personal business spread throughout the church."

"Blessed is the man that makes the Lord his trust..."
Psalm 40:4

"Yeah, I see what you mean. I don't blame

you. People do talk and your stuff will be all over."

"Sometimes it gets hard for him too. The other day he said, 'Man baby maybe I'm shooting blanks.'"

"Tell him God will put the bullets in at the right time" She said. "We don't need him shootin' you up right now!"

I needed to remember that today when at work one of the van drivers asked how long I had been married.

"Five years."

"How many children do you have?" Why do people always ask, and why do I always feel that I owe them an answer. I held out my fingers and made a zero.

"What's the matter, your husband *shootin' blanks*?" There's that statement again! I think I want to shoot him right now! I stopped myself from cursing and pushed away the unuttered, ungodly thoughts.

"I know you are joking, but it's not funny." I said nothing further on the matter and though I wanted to bolt, we continued to talk about other things.

> "...They don't know that I go **running** home when I fall down.
> They don't know who picks me up when no one is around.
> I drop my sword and cry for just awhile. 'Cause deep inside this armor the warrior is a child..." —**Twila Paris**

Thank God for every discourager, there has been an encourager. In October of 1994, I met the national founders of our non profit organization. Kimee was opening another chapter and since I was her friend I was elected to drive them around.

"So, how is your little girl?" I asked.

At the conference I'd seen her carrying around a little girl less than a year old. I thought it was odd for her to have a child that young because I knew they were in their forties.

"She's with my mother. And she's the joy of our lives. She is our only child, and we're hoping God will bless us with more."

"Really," I said, quite surprised.

"We were married seven years before I became pregnant with our son who died a few days after childbirth. I was devastated. I couldn't understand why I was being tormented this way. The agony was even more unbearable as year after year we waited for our next child."

I felt her pain.

"Seven years after my son died I got pregnant with my daughter. We waited fourteen years for her."

"Fourteen years." I said aloud. I don't know how she made it. Surely Lord you would never make me wait that long!

"I want more children. I just hope the Lord doesn't make me wait another seven years for the next one!" She laughed. "I struggled with feelings of severe grief and devastation and I felt so alone as all around me I watched other women get pregnant. I wondered how God could be so cruel to me after all I'd done for Him. It took a long, long time for me to get over that. Eventually I did and started the process of waiting again. Finally my daughter was born, but I still didn't breathe easy until she was home."

If they'd had children then, would they have had the time to dedicate themselves to such a major endeavor as this national non-profit? Would they possess their current depth and empathy to understand and feel the hurts of others?

"Wait on the Lord: be of good courage, and He shall strengthen your heart: wait I say, on the Lord..."
Psalm 27:14

I started wondering about God's barren servants in the Bible. There always seemed to be an appointed time for children. I took comfort in this thought, trusting that your birth would be according to God's plan.
God will order your footsteps and you will fulfill your purpose.

Love Mommy

CHAPTER 2

Will Somebody Please Hand Me a Stinkin' Umbrella!

"...beloved, we are confident of better things concerning you, yes, things that accompany salvation...God is not unjust to forget your work and labor of love, which you have shown toward His name...imitate those who through faith and patience inherit the promises. For when God made a promise to Abraham, because he could swear by no one greater, he swore by himself, saying, 'Surely blessing I will bless you, and multiplying I will multiply you.'...after he had patiently endured, he obtained the promise."
Hebrews 6: 9-15

February, 1996

Dear Children:

> The rain fell down
> on my windowpane
> And I could see the rain
> Just as plain
> As if the window wasn't there
> Pitter Patter
> Pitter Patter
> The rain whispered in my ear
> Then the thunder gave a ROAR!
> Jealous
> Because the rain came
> Knocking at my door
>
> It roared loud
> But I had nothing to fear
> For pretty soon
> The rain stopped
> Whispering in my ear

When I wrote these words at age thirteen I never realized how profound they were.

I was intensely afraid of Tornados because of what had happened in Xenia. Every time a storm came I had to remind myself that it was temporary and would eventually end. Sometimes I wonder what happened to my childlike faith — that faith that knows God can do ANYTHING!

Ivan, my dog, is walking around the sides of the bed trying to scratch his back. It's so funny, he thinks he's human. Now he's trying to lick the light bulb in the lamp. Dumb dog, he's going to burn his tongue. But he reminds me to trust in God, you know. He never worries about how he will get fed, or watered. He totally knows that we are going to take care of him.

So when another cycle came and went in January I had peace, because God reminded me about the God of my youth. The ONE I trusted in when my parents were fighting, when the lights where turned off, and when we didn't know if there would be food on the table. God took care of us then, and He will take care of us now.

I got angry with God though because I felt as if He wasn't hearing any of my prayers. We've been praying about the neighbor's drug activity for three years, and children now for five. I yelled, **"God, You said if we delight ourselves in You, You would give us the desires of our heart. Why can't I just get one prayer answered? Why can't I get one desire of my heart? Why can't You deal with the things that trouble ME most?"**

*"Let not your heart be troubled, you believe in God believe also in me. In my father's house are many mansions. If it were not so I would have told you. I go to prepare a place for you."—***John 14:1-2**

You see, it seemed the more we prayed about the situation across the street the worse it got! I once found an empty wine bottle in my yard and got so angry that I picked it up and threw it back across the street. It landed on the sidewalk and shattered all over it. I had become bitter in my anger.

"Do you feel any better?" Your daddy asked.

"No, but it's a good thing there aren't any more or the next one will land in their bedroom window."

"You need to calm down."

He doesn't mind a question now and then, even if we wonder why... — **4Him**

"Why is He laying all these burdens on me? You said that You would not lay on us any more than we are able to bear. I'm not that strong! I can't take it anymore!"

"Are you talking to me or God?"

"I'm talking to anyone who's listening!"

Shortly after mom called to sing me some song she'd made up, and share some weird dream she'd had. She read me a scripture and said,

"Marie don't you worry you are going to have children, so womb lineup with the Word of God!" I'm not really sure what that meant, but it made me feel better.

"Mom I know your faith is strong and you love God and believe He can do anything especially the impossible, but I'm tired."

"We all get tired baby, but you can't give up on God 'cause He ain't through with you. You gone have children, 'cause I have prayed for you to have a little girl JUST LIKE YOU!" she laughed.

I think she's trying to punish me. Even still, how can she know something that sometimes even I question?

Like last year when one day I was at work in the restroom crying and I felt the Lord saying, "*Trust Me, I am faithful and will do what I promised.*" Fifteen minutes later one of the church elders passed my office, turned around and asked how I was doing.

"I'm doing great," I say. (What a lie!)

"The thing you've been praying about for years, God says He's going to do but you've just got to keep on believing. Don't get discouraged just keep on trusting God."

"Then they cry unto the Lord in their trouble, and He brings them out of their distresses. He makes the storm calm, so that the waves thereof are still. Then they are glad because they are quiet; so He brings them into their desired haven."
Psalm 107: 28-30

"What?" I stammer, wondering if he knows what it is I've been praying about.

"I don't know when it's going to happen, but it's going to happen soon." *There's that word again.* "Don't try to do it yourself, rather let Him do it…I can't say exactly when it's going to happen, but I do know God's going to do it. Don't let anything steal your faith. Amen!"

"Uh, Amen," I nodded, while fighting to hold back the tears, because I really didn't know how to respond. But I'm wondering how did he know?

"Mother Lena by faith," his wife said a few days later.

"God revealed to my husband your problem and he began praying for your family last week." Still, the cynic in me wondered how they knew.

From that day on she began address me as, *Mother Lena by faith*. I wasn't sure how to take that. I don't like it when she calls me that around other people.

You know, it's funny, the grace of God though, and how it often works, because for every up, there is a down, for every high a there is a low, and every for mountain a valley. I got in an argument with Alisa. She and her husband accused us being jealous of them. She stated emphatically that God hasn't blessed us with children because we have some secret sin in our lives! The old Lena, would have punched her. That hurt!

"Yeah man, can you believe they really think we are that jealous? I can't believe they are tripping like that, not even calling us when their son was born!"

"Man, that's too bad we had to find out through somebody else. That's pretty insulting!"

"I know! Remember how excited we were for them? Why would they think we had suddenly changed? We're not so desperate for children that we would despise someone else."

"I know," your daddy said. "I can't understand how people can be so callous and accusatory. If sin is the reason we're not conceiving then no one should have kids. What makes their *sin* more acceptable than ours? What makes them think they are more worthy to receive kids than us?"

Talk about DOWNS!!!

Early the next morning your daddy roused me from my sleep.

"Lena, wake up! Did you hear that?"

"Hear what?"

"Gunshots!"

"Go back to sleep. We've heard gunshots coming from over there before and I'm sure we'll hear them again and nothing's ever wrong. Gunshots on this street, *nothing new*." I said groggily.

"No, this time it's different. I can feel it."

"Ok, you're a Jedi Knight now!" I laugh half asleep. "I can feel it!" I said in my best Luke Skywalker voice. "Go back to sleep."

"I'm serious! Wake up!"

As I rubbed the sleep from my eyes I knew he was right. I could feel it too. I quickly joined him at the window and surveyed what I could of the gruesome scene. There was shouting, screaming, and cursing. Fear was in the air and the theater of death was closing the curtain upon another life.

While my friend was accusing me of being jealous of the new life she'd brought into the world, I was in the uncomfortable position of consoling another mother in the loss of the life she'd birthed. I was jealous of neither of them. Talk about LOWS!"

All this living and dying reminds me of you dear children.

The day after all this stuff your uncle Jimmy came over, to ask if your daddy would attend a baby shower. He thought he would lose *man points* if he went to one.

"Well you are going to lose some more because we've decided to do the same thing when we have kids."

"How is that going by the way?"

"No problem." I answer, wondering why I always feel compelled to lie.

"What are you seeing a specialist or something? Did Horace take the sperm test? You know there might be something wrong with his sperm?" He smirked.

"No, we're not really comfortable with the whole masturbating to a porno magazine thing."

"That's how they do it?"

"As far as I know, I mean I know some people take their spouses in with them."

"There's nothing wrong with going to see a specialist." He said.

"I didn't say there was." I really didn't want to talk about it anymore, so I said, "Well I am seeing a specialist."

"Oh yeah, what's his name?" he asked

"Dr. Jesus."

"Oh yeah," he queries, "Is he good?"

"The best."

"Where is he located?"

"He has offices all over."

"How long has he been practicing?"

"Since forever!"

"How did you find out about him?"

"He came highly recommended."

Jimmy is a little deaf so by now I figured he didn't hear me when I said Dr. Jesus. I finally had to explain to him that I was talking about God.

"Oh," then jokes. "Tell Horace to quit wearing briefs." I say nothing, hoping he would get the point and end the conversation.

"You know you can always adopt." Not this again!

"Jimmy, God is totally in control and our children will come in God's time. It's simply not our time yet."

"I guess you're right." He agreed. I don't know if he really understood, or if he just wanted to shut me up.

Talk about VALLEYS!

> *"Wherefore seeing we also are compassed about with so great a cloud of witnesses, let us lay aside every weight…and run with patience the race that is set before us."* **Hebrews 12:1**

This scripture keeps me sane and keeps me from bashing the next person who suggest that *my husband wear boxers*, or *we can always adopt*, or *you might be stopping your blessing because of sin*, or *be patient*, or *take my kids*, or *you need to have more faith*, or *pray more, fast more, go to church more*…because the list goes on.

This scripture reminds me that this affliction pales in comparison to those saints who were sawn in two, fed to lions, imprisoned, and left destitute; saints who prayed for wars to end and famines to cease; saints who endured the cruelty of the slave trade, slavery, and institutional racism. They endured seeing something greater than their present suffering. And in my thoughts I honor them by holding onto the promise that God also has something better for me. I quote this scripture to remind myself that when I have nothing left to say, God has already said it all, *"Trust Me, I have not forgotten you!"*

Love Mommy

"...Write the vision, and make it plain upon the tables, that he may run that reads it. ...the vision is yet for an appointed time, but at the end it shall speak, and not lie: though it tarry, wait for it; because it will surely come..."—Habakkuk: 2:1-3

April 5, 1996

Dear Children:

Though you tarry, I will wait for you. I won't allow *anything to shake my vision. (Luke 22:31)..*

I wondered if I was on the right track. Remember those downs, lows and valleys of last month? It got worse when my brother's baby died at birth. As I struggled to deal with his death it became so easy to lose faith.

What if that happens when our children are born? Will I have the faith to believe God could raise them from the dead? Why didn't I have enough faith to believe that God could raise Joshua? Why didn't I try? If I don't have enough faith to believe that, how can I believe that God will put life into my body?

Questions, questions, questions, all I had were questions and no answers. Yet, deep down inside of me somewhere was still that tiny little mustard seed from which great faith springs. Even during my lack of understanding, I tried to make my sister-in-law feel better.

"I know that I will never fully know, nor understand your grief, but I can empathize with you. Coming on my cycle month after month is somewhat like losing a child, only it happens over, and over, and over. You start out each month with a renewed sense of hope and expectation; build yourself up for the reward, only to be crushed by the weight of its departure."

"I never thought about it like that before. How do you deal with it? I mean, in the shower this morning I just couldn't stop crying."

"I've had those shower cries too. I can't explain it, but somehow I remember God's goodness and faithfulness and I know He will bring me through."

"I just feel like I'm in a bad dream, a storm and that eventually I'll wake up. When I do wake up I'm still in the storm."

"I know," I said, "though it won't necessarily help you feel better right away, God will send others to encourage and strengthen you and to keep the flame burning. Sometimes it's only a flicker, but it will be enough."

"Do people ever say stupid stuff to you thinking they are helping?" Dana asked.

"Like what?"

"Like, '*Well at least you guys can try again to have another one.*'

I can't believe people say that. It's as if they don't realize what I have been through. I carried this life inside me for nine months and now it's gone. I carried my child, my dreams and now he's gone and people think he can be replaced!"

"They don't understand and many of them really think they are helping. But they are only making things worse. They are totally clueless."

"I just wish they wouldn't say anything at all, you know. Don't try to give me alternatives and don't try to explain it all away by saying stupid stuff like, '*God needed another flower in His garden.*' What is that about? My child is not a flower to be plucked up at someone's whim."

"I hear you, because if one more person tells me to go adopt some kids to get over my infertility I'm telling you I'm gonna catch a case!"

"Girl I ain't heard that one in a long time," she laughed.

"I mean for real, sometimes you just feel like punching people and telling them to get out of your face. A friend of mine accused me of being jealous of her because she had four kids. Can you believe that?"

"You're kidding?"

"We even have friends who are scared to tell us they are pregnant."

"Get out!"

"I guess they think I'm going to fall into some depressive state and start using drugs or something. I don't need their protection or their pity, just their love and support."

"Man, I had no idea you guys had been through all that!"

"I mean I can not imagine what it would feel like to endure your storm," I said. "But I just wanted to tell you I feel your pain. I mean especially in light of my circumstances. If I had gone all this time trying to get pregnant, and then lost the baby, I would be straight manic! I just wanted you to know I'm there for you if you need to talk."

Maybe she felt better, but I still didn't. I started to have fears; fear that complications would arise during my pregnancy, fear of miscarriage, fear that I would be waiting forever. Fear that in waiting I would lose faith. Fear that my period would come and I would have to start all over again! But if God is the Father of mercies and a God of all comfort. Then why am I so afraid?

Finally there was the fear of uncertainty because I believed God didn't want me to go to doctors anymore to have this situation investigated. But what if I am wrong? Haven't I wasted enough time? God uses doctors and he put them here for us, and has equipped them with the knowledge to heal the infirmities of mankind, so why shouldn't I go to them?

Like Habakkuk, I will stand upon my watch to see what God will say to me. I will encourage others, and I will write the vision, and make it plain upon the table, that he may run that reads it. *"For the vision is yet for an appointed time, but at the end it shall speak, and not lie: though it tarry, wait for it; because it will surely come, it will not tarry."*

NOW FAITH: *The faith you have right at this very moment!*
I never pictured my life without children. I still don't, can't. Why does it seem that the people who want kids the most can't have them?
You gave us this love Lord. Why did you give it to us if you do not intend to give us anyone to pass this it on to?"

O' Lord! What would I do without the hope that is to be found only in you? I thank you for NOW FAITH that means believing that miracles and blessings were not reserved only for those we read about

"And she was in bitterness of soul, and prayed to the Lord and wept in anguish."
I Samuel 1:10

in the Bible, people of yesterday, but that the promises of God are still in effect. NOW FAITH is the substance (*ground, matter*) of things hoped for: children, dreams, etc. NOW FAITH itself is the evidence of things not seen.

NOW FAITH is the hope I have right at this very moment! I have it right now. I stand on this NOW FAITH, no matter what I see.
I stand on it, despite my past record.

I stand upon this NOW FAITH because I know that God's reputation is at stake. His reputation has preceded time. His reputation has preceded my present sorrow. His reputation declares that He will work in this situation exceedingly. NOW FAITH declares that He did it for Hannah and He will do it for me! (*Samuel chapter 1 and Hebrews11, 12:1-5*).

"God, help Your people who are struggling with this same trial. Equip us with NOW FAITH! Hear our cry, and attend unto our prayers. You know us all by name and of our anguish and pain. You have brushed every tear from our face and comforted us when tears would no longer fall. Allow us to be joyful mothers and fathers of children. Touch us in a new and special way that we may feel the flutter of life inside, know the kick of the foot against our stomachs or a hand in our rib cage. Lord I know You can do it, only help us to have NOW FAITH to believe You will. Lord, I believe in You, and in the power of Your NOW FAITH!

Love Mommy

"Every word of God is sure: He is a shield unto them that put their trust in Him."
Proverbs 30: 5

September 30th, 1996

Dear Children:

My boss came to work and burst into my office beaming.
"I was communing with the Lord and He told me, *'Lena's pregnant.'* You're pregnant!" I looked at her funny. "Are you embarrassed?"

I didn't answer her, but I didn't know why. I guess I just didn't want anyone questioning me. How could I explain to them that the Lord had told someone else I was pregnant, yet He had failed to share this information with me or my husband? Wouldn't God tell us first? Is this a lack of faith on my part, or something else? Then I pushed the thoughts away because I didn't know what else to do with them.

Like a fool at my friend's Bridal shower, I told her mother I might be pregnant because she asked me when I was going to have children.

I didn't want to feel left out again, like something was wrong with me. I still didn't want it spread abroad, *just in case,* so I asked her to keep quiet. I must confess it felt kind of good for a minute to be able to say I was pregnant. For once, even if it was only for a few minutes, I got to feel what it was like to be special.

Later that day I debated whether or not to buy tampons. I bought them and it was a good thing too because by Monday morning I wasn't feeling so special. By then I was taking Tylenol for the cramps and ended up taking off work because I was drained and I didn't feel like having another conversation about my faith.

I recall the story of a Christian man whose daughter got sick and died. At the funeral someone said to him, "'your daughter died because you and your wife did not have enough faith.'

'Were you praying for my daughter?' The man asked.

'Why yes,' the other replied.

'Then why wasn't your faith enough?'"

That's exactly what happened when I went to work and had to explain to my boss that I was not pregnant.

"Well it must be your fault, I know we heard God!"

"What! God forbid you could've been wrong. Or maybe you really didn't hear anything at all. Maybe you just said some stuff so you could seem spiritually superior."

"How could you say that to me?" She was upset.

I can say a lot of things when I am pissed, I thought to myself. My mind was ready to burst at the seams as one million thoughts fought to exit my brain. Like crab-lice in my mind, each thought was crawling on top of the other in a desperate attempt to escape the madness going on inside my head. Finally one thought did escape-how does she really know so much about my problem anyway?

So I got to thinking, maybe that's what happened with me? I hadn't talked to anyone but Bonita and she and her husband were also good friends with my boss and her husband? I had a sudden epiphany, "Oh my God, Bonita sold me out!" The one person I thought I could trust had sold my confidence. I resolved in my heart not to confide in anyone again.

I prayed, *"Lord No more words of "divine revelation" that did not come from You. We've got enough troubles on our hands without trying to sort through foolishness."*

"In You O Lord do I put my trust, let me never be ashamed..."
Psalms 31:1-3

Recently I heard a message entitled, *Living in the Land of AND*. It was about being beaten down with **_anxiety_**, **_bad news_**, **_discouragement_**, and **_depression_**. God is willing to give us the reward if we will turn **_anxiety_** into **_anticipation_**, **_bad news_** into **_never giving up_**, and **_discouragement_** and **_depression_** into **_deliverance,_** is what the speaker said.

This is our Red Sea hour–to mockers and to the enemy it seems as if God has forsaken us and failed us. However, this is exactly where God wants us to be, for it is in this very place where He will show Himself strong.

> *"Our difficulties are but God's challenges, and many times He makes them so hard that we must get above them or go under...*
> *We are pushed by the very emergency into God's best."*
> A.B. Simpson

Mrs. Charles Cowan tells the story of a woman who was going through a great trial. In the midst of it she felt that God had forsaken her.

One evening after a prayer meeting she said, *"God and I have been very wonderful friends, but He seems to have withdrawn Himself from me. I seem to be utterly left alone."* Then looking off in the distance, and with tears she continued, *"But if I never see His face again, I will keep looking at the spot where I saw His face last."*

Thus we are pushed by the emergency of our ills into being better people and therefore we also will keep our faces turned to the place where we last saw Him.

"When we feel cast down Lord remind us that we are not forsaken. Remember those of us who long for a baby and who cry out to You in desperation. Hold us and help us know that You are as close to us as the air we breathe, because You are the air we breathe."

Love Mommy

CHAPTER 3

Year of Jubilee is the Year of Grief To Me

"Praying always with all prayer and supplication in the spirit..."
Ephesians 5:18a

February 19, 1997

Dear Children:

The other day, after watching our niece and nephew, your father and I asked ourselves, "do we really want kids?" They wanted to play and we wanted to watch a movie. Shoot, we'd pretty much gotten used to doing things when we wanted to do them. Was I really ready to give up myself? Now not only do I believe I can wait on God; I want to wait on Him.

At least that's what I told myself in January.

I am no longer feeling jubilant. I feel like those saints in despair who have no choice but to fully rely on God. Charles Spurgeon said that great hearts can only be made by great troubles. He further said:

"When the night lowers and the tempest is coming on, the Heavenly Captain is always closest to His crews. It is a blessed thing that when we are most cast down, then it is that we are most lifted up by the consolations of the Spirit."

My tempest started with a light period and I was told this could mean you are pregnant. Convinced by a friend, I drove to a place I'd heard about on the radio that provides counseling and free pregnancy testing. I was nervous and anxious, not about what I thought the test might reveal, but rather by what it wouldn't reveal, even though the Bible says we should be anxious for nothing.

I walked through the door feeling very much like an 18 year old who'd just been knocked up by her boyfriend, rather than the 30 year old professional that I was. After filling out a short form, I was led into a room by a counselor who asked for my name and address. I wondered what she needed to know all that for. I gave her our old address. She asked me my birthday and I wondered what my birthday has to do with anything? Forgive me Lord, but I lied. Then she wanted to know how I'd heard about the place as well as my views on abortion.

All this for a pregnancy test! I should have just bought one. I know the lady was just doing her job, and she was really nice, but good grief, if I really were an 18-year-old hiding from my parents I would have run right out the door.

Finally, she gave me the cup and I spilled some pee on the floor while filling it. It was embarrassing!

I cleaned it up, washed my hands, cleaned off the jar, and carried it back. She gave me the test and instructions. When I realized I had to do it myself I looked at her like, "Okay you can leave now." She didn't, so I proceeded to administer it. We made uncomfortable small talk while waiting for the results.

"So...how are you doing?"

"Fine," I replied, wishing she wouldn't talk to me.

"What do you do for a living?"

"I'm a Substance Abuse Prevention Specialist." Stop talking!

"Really? That sounds interesting. What exactly do you do?"

"I work with kids and their parents. I design and implement programs to help them stay off drugs."

"Wow, that's pretty neat. I imagine that can get pretty wild and stressful?"

"Yeah, it makes for some interesting days."

"So, is there anything in your life that could be causing you stress?"

"We're moving." I answered uncomfortably. Then it hit me; perhaps I could be under stress. I just never thought it was possible, but it could've been. Hey, I did live across the street from drug dealers, and next door to a bunch of dope heads. For the past few years I had been dealing with job related issues. No wonder I couldn't get pregnant. Maybe the stress is interfering with my cycle. It's not the first time it's happened!"

After four long minutes the buzzer rang. I acted like I didn't hear it because I didn't want to know what the results were.

"Negative." She said.

"I can see that."

"I encourage you to see a doctor anyway."

"There is no point in that." I tried not to look at her.
"Well come back anytime." She was nice, but I don't think so.

I wanted to cry, but maintained my cool. I wanted to run, but maintained my composure. I politely said goodbye and exited the building as fast as I could.

My reaction to the negative pregnancy test confirmed that the words I'd uttered all month never really reached the truth that lied in my heart.

I wanted children more now than I ever did before, and the realization forced me to confront my motives for wanting them. What was I really basing this desire on?

Initially I think I wanted them because I thought children would solidify our bond of marriage. But then maybe it was because everyone else expected us to have children? You know, you get married and automatically have children, right?

As an American of African descent, this expectation is magnified. People automatically expect women of color to be fertile. After all, there's the mythology of the big, black, breeding studs and "*studdettes*." We are often led to believe, even by our own people that slave women dropped babies like it was nothing and then went right back to working in the field.

The stories I'd heard as a child made me accept the lie that no slave woman ever died during childbirth, or had problems with infertility.
This smacks right in the face of survival of the race. Procreation meant the race would not die despite the horrors of slavery. Reproduction represented the slave's one hope of a bright future and expected end. We were simply too strong, *too fertile to be infertile* so to speak. Young, black, and infertile, what an oxymoron! What a lie! The reality is that black women struggle with infertility as much as any other race.

Margaret Marsh and Wanda Ronner, in their book, <u>The Empty Cradle: Infertility in America from Colonial Times to the Present,</u> provide proof that infertility was roughly the same among all races and cultures. However, for reasons unknown black women had a higher rate of childlessness than whites in the 1950's, as they had for decades...and magazines aimed at black Americans focused on the issue.

Tan Confessions, directed at working-and-middle class Americans of African descent, published several fictional accounts of infertility... and the publisher of one of the more popular books on infertility, Sam Gordon Berkow's, <u>Childless</u>, advertised the book in Ebony, which also published a number of articles on infertility *"clinics, artificial insemination, and adoption. Interest was wide-spread..."* So if I wasn't trying to prove something to my people, what was I trying to prove?

Over time I convinced myself that I wanted children so that I could raise great men and women of God, like those women in the Bible. I told myself that God wanted that from me, even if God doesn't want it, then the Christian world sure expects it of you.
"How long have you been a Christian?" They ask accusingly. "Six years? And you still don't have kids?" Their silent accusations forced me to believe that raising *little gods* was a much more noble reason for wanting kids and I felt it would make me more worthy of being a mother. So like Hannah I made promises to God. *"God if You will give me children then I promise I will give them back to You..."*

If I really love kids like I say I do, why am I so apprehensive about foster parenting or adopting? Would doing so mean I am giving up on God; that if I foster parent or adopt I don't really believe that He will allow me to have a child from my own womb?

I know most of our friends think it would be best for our emotional well being if we would just admit that our bodies have failed us.

Which leads me back to the original question of why do I want kids? And that only leads me to other questions like, if I just want kids shouldn't *anyone's* kids fulfill the maternal instinct? Do I want to have the birthing experience? Do I need to fulfill an expected womanly or cultural role? Do I want to fulfill a lifelong dream? Do I want to be immortal, have a little image of myself running around, an image connected by blood? How much do I need this child? My child? My blood child? Would I love an adopted child as much as you, <u>the child of my dreams</u>? You are my Isaac; would another child be my Ishmael?

So many things I don't know but I question, but one thing I do know–I will never trust my period again. It has lied to me before and I should not have been surprised that it had lied to me again. Still, despite the hurt, I am filled with the hope of God's words — *be fruitful and multiply*.

Love Mommy

> *"And God said, let there be lights in the firmament of the heaven...
> and let them be for signs and for seasons..."*
> **Genesis 1:14**

May 10, 1997

Dear Children:

Time belongs to God, as He is the author of it. When we are growing anxious or impatient, we need only remember that God has our days, weeks, months, and years in His hands.

The first chapter of Psalms deals with seasons. I hadn't really paid attention to that before. See it says ...*brings forth <u>his fruit</u> in <u>his season</u>...* Indicating that every tree, every plant, everything, does not come into season at the same time, nor do plants, trees, etc., bear the same fruit. I've been comparing myself to others, and I had completely forgotten that I am not the same as others. God made me a totally different way.

> *"To everything there is a season, and a time to every purpose under heaven: a time to be born and a time to die; a time to plant, and a time to pluck up that which is planted..."*
> **Ecclesiastes 3:1, 2**

My mind began to wander with meditations so I then looked up the word season and I studied Ecclesiastes 3:1-8. A season is a suitable, natural, and convenient period of time in which we are cured and/or rendered competent through trial and experience. In other words, we are becoming usable.

How could God use me to help others unless I had undergone the same trial and experience?

In Season: At the right moment, opportunity.

In God's time He'd give me the opportunity to be a mother.

Seasonable: In keeping with the time or the season. Occurring or performed at the proper time; timely. (Applies to whatever is appropriate or timely for the season.)

I wouldn't wear a winter coat in the summer nor will I bear a child until it is my time and/or season.

These scriptures brought me peace in knowing that if we obey God and keep His Word then He will bring us our prosperity (i.e. children) in our season. This prosperity could come in more than one way because every living thing produces *something*.

God encouraged me that our fruit will come in its season.

A few months after that wonderful study, I stood on the precipice of an abyss and was on the verge of sliding into it. I was poised on that volcano of destruction and ready to jump. I faced a depression so deep that life or death almost didn't matter. But somewhere in the deep recesses of my soul was an anchor that kept me from making that forward plunge into eternal darkness.

It was the strength of a God who'd experienced pain and suffering and who could understand my deep grief and relieve it.

> *"For we do not have a High Priest who cannot sympathize with our weaknesses...Let us therefore come boldly to the throne of grace, that we may obtain, mercy and find grace to help in time of need."*
> **Hebrews 4:15, 16**

In January, for a whole week before my cycle was due, I kept reminding myself not to get too excited. I distracted myself with silly thoughts like who decided it was going to be called a *period and w*ho first made the statement, 'My period is on?' Does it mean you are going to have it PERIOD, so just shut up and deal with it!

That Friday night as I lay on my bed, I began to imagine as I do, often getting too caught up. This time I imagined my baby shower and how packed it would be with my friends and family.

Finally I fell to sleep dreaming that I was rocking you to sleep while stroking the soft locks of your curls and smelling your sweet baby breath. A couple of times during the night I awoke to see if my period had started, and then I fell back to sleep dreaming of you.

I woke up that morning and checked again. Still it hadn't come. I showered, dressed, ate breakfast, and cleaned up, still no period. We were just about to sit down for family devotions, when I felt the stirrings of my old familiar *friend,* which by now I considered my foe. I excused myself and went to the bathroom to check.

I sat on the toilet, grabbed a small section of toilet paper, placed it upon my middle finger, reached up into my vagina, and wiped. I examined it and found exactly what I thought I was feeling — blood. Though it had not yet reached its final destination, I knew from experience that it would.

I sat there and scolded myself for dreaming; I had set myself up for this disappointment. I tried to stop the rising river of tears from bursting through the dam I had so carefully constructed, but it was too late. There was a weakness, caused by the innocent imaginations of my heart the night before.

My previous ruminations had caused the failing in my defenses. The pressure of those waters was building and there would be no stopping them, they would be released! Before I could think any further, I found my head drawn to the cup of my hands, and I filled them with my tears.

No matter how hard I tried I could not contain them. I didn't want your daddy to see me crying. How could I let him see how stupid I had been for letting my imaginations get the best of me? I knew I needed him, but I just couldn't let him see.

So I just sat there angry and in unbearable pain. This was a deep pain; coming from a place I had never been. Something was dying and that something was me. This was a trial of cruel mocking that made false promises to me every chance it got and thus hope, once my friend had now become my enemy.

Finally, I managed to contain the waters overflowing my heart's banks, only to have them return with greater intensity when I reached for the sanitary napkin. I shook and trembled with new tears as I opened the package I needed to stem my menstrual flow. My hands and fingers grew weak as I fit it into its place. I was sick —heartsick, and I wanted to crawl into that closet and stay there forever. I could not say to my soul, "It is enough! Stop crying."

Somehow, despite the ache, I was able to rise. A thousand thoughts crowded my mind, each one straining to burst forth all at once. I felt mocked, rejected, dismayed, and in despair. I looked at my reflection in the mirror and saw a failure. To me I'd failed as a woman in the most important way of all. To the world I seemed to have it all, but in my mind I was a piece of malfunctioning equipment ripe for the refuse. I could hear my old boyfriends saying, "Phew, I'm glad I didn't marry her, she can't even have kids." I just didn't understand what was wrong with me! With these thoughts came fresh tears, and my body wracked in anguish from the hurt.

Shaking, I washed my hands, but I couldn't go down those stairs yet. I sat drowning in a sea of self imposed pity. Between the crying was an ominous silence that spoke volumes. It was worse than the crying because in the silence thoughts came and they started a new round of weeping.

Finally, I went back to the table and as soon as daddy saw me he held out his arms and said, "Come here baby." Ivan, sensing something was amiss, pulled up alongside me. "It's going to be alright." He said. I sat on his lap and lay in his arms like a limp rag doll.

I sat there for a few more minutes then we had our devotions. I don't really remember what we read because half the time I was reading through blurred vision. Then he prayed and hugged me because he understood that I had nothing to offer. I was merely in too much pain to pray.

I know I should've turned to God, but instead I turned away.

I went upstairs, climbed in the bed, even though it was only 12 noon, and cried myself to sleep. As I cried, I found the strength to utter one simple prayer, "Lord, help me through this. Help me make it through the storm."

I awoke around three in a zombie-like state and took a shower where I cried again. I felt like someone I loved deeply had died; like I had lost my child. Who could I call that would understand? There was no one in my camp. I couldn't call Bonita; she had revealed my secret to others.

No one I knew who understood but God. He allowed himself to be compassed about with infirmity, all infirmity — *my infirmity*! He alone knew how I felt. He was after all my God, my Lord, and My Savior. He had died for me. So in my weeping I finally turned to him.

I was weak. I cried some more. *He was strong*. He picked me up. As much as I hurt, this new wave of crying was cleansing me.

This experience was creating a new me, one who could also empathize with the hurts and infirmities of others. When at last I was able to get dressed I joined daddy downstairs as he sat on the loveseat watching a movie.

"...We are troubled on every side, yet not distressed; we are perplexed but not in despair; persecuted but not forsaken; cast down but not destroyed..."
II Corinthians 4: 8-10

"Snap out of it." I heard while staring blankly at the screen. He smiled, "We are not going to have any more depression around here." Then he hugged me, "Baby, you've got to come up out of this."

"I know."

"I know, but it hurts so much."

He was trying his best to be strong for the both of us, if we both started sinking who would rescue us? We hugged for a few more minutes then he asked if I felt better. I smiled, and then went to the kitchen to fix something to eat.

Later we went to the buy Ivan some dog food. On the way we caught a few minutes of a radio broadcast entitled, *Beyond the Shadow of a Doubt*. It was about a couple struggling with infertility. They were dismayed, fearful, and ready to give up hope?

What are the odds that I would be going through what I went through on that day and be in the car at that particular time, listening to that broadcast? I was touched that God loved me enough to do that!

Before I went to bed that night I again read of Abraham and Sarah's struggles with infertility in Genesis. If anyone had a reason to doubt God it was Abraham. The man was OLD, but in his old age (weakness) God made him strong. It's when it seems the most impossible that God often moves. To be like Abraham means to trust God despite the odds.

The next morning we prepared for church though I really didn't want to go. I was still smarting from the day before and I did not want to run into Bonita or Marion. I was afraid if I saw either of them I would burst into tears. The message was on the condition of your faith.

"The evidence/unveiling of things not yet seen means that the *evidence* already existed..." the speaker said.

"How about that," I said aloud.

"There are three areas of faith;" she continued. "The faith that *sees into the future*, that's the kind that Joseph had. Then there is *faith that moves beyond feelings*. I'm sure Abraham didn't *feel* like moving. He didn't feel like offering up his son as a sacrifice, but he trusted God. And finally, there's *the faith that overcomes fear*. You don't think Abraham was afraid when told him to offer up Isaac? How would you feel?"

Do I have the faith to believe that God is handling the areas I can't control? I realized that regarding infertility the "*heat*" had been turned up and my faith was beginning to liquefy.

I would look into the *<u>future</u>* and be *<u>fearful</u>* that it would be empty and childless. I felt dead inside and hopeless. My menstrual cycle was on and I felt like nothing could ever make it stop. I felt that I would never know what it would be like to carry a child. I had to see my future with my children and overcome my fears despite how I felt.

We went to the altar for prayer and after the service ended Marion came over to encourage me. I didn't mind because we'd always felt a kinship with her and her husband. Through their struggles of parenting a special needs child, they too had learned to rely on God. We had a connection and when she called later that day I shared with her the events of Saturday.

Marion is *real people,* you know what I mean. *Real people* share their experiences with you in a way that lets you know they understand. Often, *they don't* say anything at all; knowing that nothing can make you feel any better so they simply lend an ear and offer up a heartfelt prayer. Others *over spiritualize* everything, throwing out some formula that's supposed to make everything all right.
   "*Girl, it's gonna be all right, you just gotta have MORE faith.*"
   How can you have MORE faith? You either have it or you don't.
   "*Don't worry about it, if it's meant to be, it will be.*"
   Don't want to hear that!
   "*Girl, you ain't been through nothing. Let me tell you about what I'VE been through...*"
   Don't really care!
   "*Maybe you better check yourself to be sure you don't have some secret sin or unforgiveness keeping you from getting pregnant?*"
   Secret sin, what the heck does that mean and unforgiveness, who doesn't have some.

After Marion and I talked I felt better. Through her I was reminded that God's word says:

> "*So do not fear, for I am with you; do not be dismayed, for I am your God.*
> *I will strengthen you and help you;*
> *I will uphold you with my righteous right hand.*"—**Isaiah 41:10**

Saturday I was extremely down, on the borderline of falling into a state of depression. I was ***fearful*** of the ***future*** and filled with ***doubt***. I could barely quell the flood of uncertainties quickly crowding my head, but God truly upheld me with His righteous right hand.

Love Mommy

GOD IS MY REFUGE

"Nevertheless the foundation of God stands sure, having this seal,
The Lord knows them that are his…"
2 Timothy 2:19

June 15, 1997

Dear Children:

God's presence is with me, comforting me. As a father does when his child is hurt, I picture His arms around me and I know that I am safe. He keeps back all those who would pry me from Him. *"When the enemy comes in like a flood, He lifts up a standard against them."* I can run to Him when I am hurt and my wounds are cleansed and bandaged before He lets me go, and even though I can sometimes still feel the pain, I feel the bandage and am reminded that all has been fixed and in time I will heal.

REMAIN STEADFAST

"… a certain man was there, which had an infirmity thirty and eight years. When Jesus saw him lie, and knew that he had been now a long time in that case, he said unto him, 'Will you be made whole?'…." –***John 5:1-18***

The man possessed steadfast faith; otherwise he would not have gone to that pool everyday. Jesus is Lord over time. Keep coming to the one who stills the water.

I can see it Lord, just like I was there
The sick man Waiting
For the stirring of the water…
I can see him cryin'
But he never stopped tryin'
Year after year he shed tears…still he kept on coming…people laughed
And shook their heads asking,
"Why does he keep believing?
Nothing's ever gonna happen."
But they didn't know He had a friend…
Watchin', and Oh, He could see it all
He asked, "Would you be made whole?"
How could he know he was talking to the one who stirred the water!
And…how could he disobey his authority
when he heard these words he could see
what others failed to see
He is eternity
He's the mighty Prince of Peace
He sets the captives free…
and he wouldn't let him --
die without his miracle."

HOW TO HAVE THE PEACE OF GOD

Do not be anxious about anything, but in everything by prayer and petition with thanksgiving, present your request to God. And the peace of God, which transcends all understanding, will guard your hearts and mind….
Philippians 4: 6, 7

1. Rejoice in the Lord always!
2. Let your gentleness be known to all men.
3. Be anxious for nothing, but in everything by;
4. Prayer and supplication, with thanksgiving,
5. Make your request to God.

God's peace will enter in and how you can have peace is beyond your understanding. That peace guards your mind, protecting you from unhealthy stress and emotional overload. You don't need to understand *why* anymore because you completely trust God's purpose and plan for you. That anxiety, of all the fears (real or imaginary) can only be overcome by trusting and relying on the Holy Spirit and God's provision, care, and sovereignty; and praying to Him in assurance.

GOD'S GRACE IS ENOUGH

"... 'My grace is sufficient for you, for my power is made perfect in weakness.' ...For when I am weak, then am I strong."
II Corinthians 12:9, 10

Sufficient: As much as is needed. Enough. Adequate.

Grace: Unmerited (*undeserved and undetermined*) favor. Divine love and protection bestowed freely upon mankind. Protected and/or sanctified by the power of God. An excellent source or power granted by God.

I read in the *Word in Life Study Bible* that, "*weakness has a way of making us rely on God for more than our strengths. What weakness in your life might God desire to use for His purposes?*"

So do not fear, for I am with you; do not be dismayed, for I am your God. I will strengthen you and help you: I will uphold you with my righteous right hand.
Isaiah 41:10

He is THE LORD GOD MY STRENGTH–my foundation, the one on whom I can safely build.

He is my refuge, the person in whom I can find safety and protection. Though this deeper relationship was birthed in heartfelt pain, the reward of growing closer to God is sweet. I once heard someone say that in order to savor the sweet scent of roses you must first work your way around the thorns.

"In the Lord I put my trust, how can you say to my soul, 'Flee as a bird to your mountain."—**Psalm 11**

So, what can I say about this great God
that has not already been said?
What more could I say of His mercy
or of the lives brought back from the dead?
If I dared to speak of the refuge
one can find under His wings,
who would really take out the time
to seriously contemplate these things?
So what more can I say of this great God
who means more than words could express?
Even the pen in my hand cannot adequately impress
Just how much the Lord means you see–
I feel I cannot do justice with this
grace that's sufficient for me!

"Lord, You have been our dwelling place in all generations. Before the mountains were brought forth, or ever, you have formed the earth and the world, even from everlasting to everlasting, you are God. So teach us to number our days; that we may gain a heart of wisdom."
Psalm 90: 1, 2

Love Mommy

CHAPTER 4

TKO: Trusting God When You're Getting A Beat Down!

November 10, 1998

Dear Children:

I faced a moral conflict as I gazed upon the photo of the woman carrying her child through the rising floodwaters. I grieved for her poverty and circumstance, while at the same time envying her for being able to feel something I could not feel, the bond of love between a mother and her child. How do you reconcile this mindset?

Who would ever believe that I struggle with these feelings? The reality is that infertility is like a plague that infects my mind, so much so that most people will never know the inner pain and hopelessness I tussle with.

> *"They became His temple, and their hearts are a holy of holies in which His blessed Presence abides. From that central citadel He works, enduring the man who has received Him with power…"*—**Sallie Chesam**

I have learned though, that our life is a Bible in progress and God cares about every aspect of it, big and small. The people in the Bible were ordinary people, just like you and me. They were placed in *extraordinary* circumstances and their faith in God allowed them to accomplish *extraordinary* things, and as a result they received *extraordinary* blessings. At the time they didn't realize the significance of the *ordinary* trust they had in their Creator. As I write God reminds me of the ordinary occasions.

Like when we didn't have money for our honeymoon, we prepared to go anyway and God provided. Lela my mom's friend started planning her wedding years before she even had a boyfriend. Don't you know that woman got a good man a few years later!

What about when my mom bought a house when she had no, money, no down payment, and bad credit! The owners paid her closing cost and a special lending program paid her down payment. I still don't know how she got around the bad credit thing, but God made a way.

A few years later, God did the same thing for us by providing resources and funds from seemingly thin air for your daddy to finish school

These were all *seemingly ordinary events happening to ordinary people.*

"The Lord is my strength and my song."
Psalm 118:14

So, you be *strong in the Lord and in the power of His might* so you can endure what's coming. Know where you stand, and know that God always has your back.

So in reconciling my earlier mindset I understand that it's okay if I have conflicting thoughts as I am very ordinary on my own. And in my ordinary circumstance of extraordinary sorrow, God will someday, make me into a beautiful instrument of praise.

> *"For what song can there be where there is languor and fainting? What brave music can be born in an organ, which is short of breath? There must first be strength if we would have fine harmonies. And so the good Lord comes to the song less, and with holy power He brings the gift of saving health."* —**John Henry Jowett**

True success is faithfully following God in the places we currently find ourselves in.

"Lord fill our lives with the music of praise and thanksgiving to You. We are ordinary people who have agreed to trust you to do extraordinary things in our lives. Let our very lives be a melody of Your grace and goodness. May the music of Your Holy Spirit flow in and from the lives of our children; that every life they touch would feel the power, presence, and praise of Your Spirit. Let this prayer be a source of strength that leads the dry soul to You."

Love Mommy

"...There are three things that are never satisfied, four never say, enough! The grave, the barren womb, the earth that is not satisfied with water–And the fire never says, enough!"—***Proverbs 30:15-16***

April 25, 1999

Dear Children:

I had my nerve, giving this speech to my laid off co-workers about trusting God and our steps being ordered by Him, blah, blah, blah. Oh I really impressed everyone, EXCEPT GOD! On the way home I heard a voice ask, "You know, if you really believe that your steps are ordered by God, why were you in the bathroom crying earlier?"

What could I say? What answer can you give when God asks you a question like that? I was speechless.

The day started out well you know. See I was on my way to work and I was feeling on top of the world. I'm jamming, you know, listening to Fred Hammond's, *"No Way"*-a song about praising God in the midst of your troubles.

> *"Woke up to the sound of morning news, lookin' out the window, things is cool, checkin' on my list of things to do, and everything's okay.* (My day at work started exactly like this.) *Telephone rings and then I learn, my life tries to take a drastic turn, my world tries to cave in, do you hear me, before 10 AM, but No Way you won't lose..."*

It goes on to talk about how God reassures us that He is in control of every aspect of our lives, and we will win the battle against our enemies, no matter who or what they are. God's armor will protect us from the blows designed to pummel us. Powerful words huh, I never knew they'd challenge me before the day ended.

I heard the phone ring in Missy's office, and she started screaming for joy.

"Lena I'm getting ready to transfer a call to you," she said after hanging up her phone. "Well really it's for everybody, but I think you'll really appreciate it."

"What is everyone getting a raise and I got a bigger bonus?" I wondered aloud. That would be cool! I continued checking my messages.

"Hi guys," it started. "This is Rick and Jackie. We just called to see what you will be doing the day after Christmas."

"Hopefully going on a cruise to the Bahamas at your expense," I said. The nature of the question was so strange that surely it must be leading up to something like that.

But then Missy's happy squeal and Rick's excited tone confirmed what the sinking, sick feeling in my heart had already told me. I began to feel like a boxer who'd just gone the distance and doesn't have much strength left. He's been fighting a good fight and up until the last round the contest is a draw, and suddenly his opponent launches a *one, two, and three-punch combination*. Bam, one to the jaw! Bzam, one to the chin! Bdam, one right in the center of the stomach!

You wonder where they got the strength and why you didn't see it coming because you thought you were about to take him out, and instead he's taking you down. I was crying. They were having a baby and wanted to thank us all for praying and ask that we keep her in our prayers. There was nothing wrong with that.

I don't remember what else he said, because like the fighter I was going down! My vision was blurry and my knees were buckling and I was struggling to maintain my balance. I wondered why she would think that I above all others was supposed to be so happy.

Oh, I knew why, because they were praying for me and in her own way she was trying to encourage me. Why was I so surprised and so unguarded, it wasn't as if I hadn't prayed for them. She'd had major heart surgery two years ago and doctors weren't sure if her heart could handle the strain of pregnancy. Last month they'd gotten the okay from her doctor and just like that she was pregnant!

I cried. I was tempted with *jealousy*. I yelled inside my head to God in *anger*, "WHAT'S GOING ON LORD?" I know they suffered when they were young, but now it seems like they have it all. They get whatever they want, and everything seems so easy for them. Couldn't they have to fight for one thing now?"

I cried in *sorrow* and *despair*, "I've been praying for nine years for my child. I pray for her and she gets pregnant in less than a month!

I'm going down for the count. I know I am wrong for the way I feel.

Still, I can feel the mat on my fingertips, on my knuckles, on my palms, when suddenly some deep reservoir of hope appears and I take it like a thirsty man in the desert! I don't know where it comes from, and I can't explain it, but suddenly I hear Fred Hammond saying to me, "***No way, no way, you won't lose…***" I begin to rise. I push myself up from that mat. I remember the lyrics, and though I'm not mighty yet, I softly begin to sing, "I hear You Lord, reassuring me…" and somehow, some way, I know I won't lose.

> *"…I am easily discouraged by the silence of God, when my prayers do not seem to be answered, I am tempted to give up, and not ask again. I identify more readily with the wavering man who declared to Jesus, 'I do believe; help me overcome my unbelief…'* —**Phillip Yancey**, Author

It's funny how faith appears when you least expect it. Romans 10:17 declares that faith comes by hearing, and hearing by the word of God. I hear that song in my head and I'm able to rise. Trying times will come, but I pray that God will help us to accept our adversity with humility.

Instead of asking *why* Lord, may we ask *what* is it You want to teach us through this. Let us be teachable in our present situation and grow closer to You as a result.

"You have a soul diseased. Put it into the hand of the Great Physician! Trust Him and He will take care of it. He has had some of the most hopeless cases. He was able to heal all that came to Him while on earth. He is the same today." — D.L. Moody

When mom was in the hospital recuperating from her first surgery I dreamed she was walking through the darkness. It was pitch black on every side of her, as if she was in the middle of a forest clearing. There was darkness behind her and much more before her, but in the center of the darkness where she was there was bright, shining light.

Two giant angels walked beside her, one on each side. Jesus, from the shadows was watching it all. I felt like God was telling me that mom has come out of a great darkness, but there was more to come, but that we could be at peace knowing that He was/is always there guiding her and comforting her.

In that same spirit we can trust that God will guide us and comfort us during our dark hours. He may not illuminate our past or future, but our present path will always be well lit. No way, no way, we won't lose.

We can trust Him, even when we're getting a beat down.

Love Mommy

CHAPTER 5

When the Clouds Move—
Faith Appears!

"Now Solomon the son of David was strengthened in his kingdom, and the Lord his God was with him and exalted him exceedingly…"
II Chronicles 1-3

September 9, 2000

Dear Children:

January I went to a female doctor referred by Kimee for my annual exam. I thought a woman might be more sensitive to me regarding our struggle with infertility. Without discussing things she said, "I'll write a prescription for you to take to Miami Valley Fertility Clinic to have your husband's sperm tested, then after that we can talk some more." That was it? No discussion about what I've been through, possible reasons for infertility? Maybe that was her style, but after everything I'd already endured I expected a little more compassion.

After the exam I said, "I'm having a lot of pain right in here," as I pointed to the area where I knew my ovaries were located.

"Oh, it's normal to have some pain around there," she shrugged her shoulders nonchalantly.

"Are you sure, because it really hurts?"

"Yeah, it's perfectly normal to have pain there around your monthly."

"But it's not just during my cycle that I have pain."

"Well it's normal to have pain two weeks prior due to hormonal fluctuations." She said.

"Yeah, but I hurt all the time, not just around my cycle. One of my previous doctors said I had small ovarian cysts. Maybe they've gotten bigger and that's what's causing the pain?"

"Trust me, it's not a problem. It's normal."

"Perhaps you could schedule an ultrasound just to be sure?" I asked.

"I don't think that's necessary," she was becoming irritated.

"I'd really feel a lot better if you would. I'd also like you to schedule a mammogram just to double-check my breast tissue. It's really fibrous and I normally have a biannual mammogram as an added precaution."

"You don't need a mammogram or an ultrasound, but if it will make you feel better," she said obviously annoyed by my insistence,

"I'll have my office schedule one." I was upset by her lack of concern for my issues and the source of my pain.

Later I spoke to Kimee about it and she gave me the name of yet another doctor. I told her she was already two for two in sending me to stupid, unsympathetic doctors, but she was insistent.

"Lena, I promise you this one is great! I never went to the other doctors, but this one I know personally. If it wasn't for him neither I, nor Ulysses would be here."

"What are you talking about Kimee?"

"Remember I told you about the car accident I was in during college and how it messed up my back?"

"Oh, yeah."

"When I went into labor my doctor wanted me to have a C- section because of my spine and the fact that Ulysses was so big due to the gestational diabetes. I refused because during that time some woman's babies had their fingers cut off during their C-sections and I was so afraid that was going to happen to Ulysses. Plus, I was afraid the medicine would put me out and someone would kidnap my baby."

"Girl you are crazy." I said laughing.

"I know, but I had been in labor for nearly 24 hours, so I am sure I wasn't thinking straight. I was scared. Anyway the stupid doctor told me, 'Well just go ahead and die then because that's what's going to happen if you don't let me take this baby.' I was so mad. He refused to deliver my baby if I didn't do it his way. He dropped me and another lady that same day. Her baby died."

"Oh my God!"

"It just happened with me that Doctor Watson was also on call that night and he took over the case. He told me he'd give me a few more hours, but after that they would have to do what they had to do. I loved his demeanor right off. I still wasn't letting him take my baby though."

"I don't know girl, the last two doctors you recommended…"

"I know, but I'm telling you he is different. He is awesome! He's up in Yellow Springs and you know them women are not going to let any doctor deliver their babies unless they believe he is the best."

"That's true."

"I promise you, he saved our lives." She continued.

"I almost died but he came right in and worked with me and delivered Ulysses natural. Now he would've done the C-section if it had come down to that, but he listened to me and gave me more time."

"Well I do need an ultrasound to check on this ovary, so I guess it won't hurt to at least get that scheduled." I was still skeptical, but in spite of my reservations I scheduled an appointment. I asked your daddy to go with me because this was our problem and we had to do this together.

"I don't know," he said hesitantly. "I thought we were going to wait until September before we really started looking into this issue and get a complete work up?"

"I know, but I have to go anyway, so we might as well use it as a preliminary opportunity to get some answers." He finally agreed.

Immediately upon meeting Dr. Watson we both felt good. We really liked his manner and his accent was cool. Though his conversation was lighthearted and cheery, his concern was genuine and his knowledge was extensive. He seemed very kind, patient, understanding and caring. Despite my reservations I was completely at ease.

"How long have you guys been married?" He asked after the general inquiry of past struggles with infertility.

"Ten years," we both replied.

"Ten years!" He exclaimed. "And you've never used birth control in all that time?"

"No," We said.

He asked us some additional related questions, and openly expressed anger at his colleague's lack of care and lamented with us over our previous struggles. He seemed especially annoyed at the last doctor I'd seen who ignored my pain.

"Are your periods painful?"

"Yes."

"Pain is never normal. Do you sometimes have nausea and vomiting with your periods?"

"Yes."

"Have you ever had to miss school or work because of the pain?"

"Yes."

"Have you ever had pain during intercourse?"

"Lot's of times," I said.

"And you are having the pelvic pain and pain around your ovaries?"

"Yes, that's right, but that's normal isn't it? That's what all the other doctors kept telling me."

"Some mild cramping around your monthly maybe, but severe pain like yours is not normal."

"It's not?"

"No, and I can't believe anyone let you go this long in this much agony."

"All this time, I thought something might be wrong, but I was always told it was normal."

"Don't worry, within two months we will have an answer to your problem. We're going to get you pregnant. Let me examine you and we'll talk some more afterwards." After the exam we went back to his office.

"Now the first step in the infertility work-up process is to have you tested, Horace I'm going to schedule you for a sperm analysis. You can take the sample at home; you just have to get it to the lab within 30 minutes." No doctor had ever told us that before.

"Technically," he continued. "You have 45 minutes, but they want it there within 30 just to be on the safe side." Then he said laughing, "Now if you get into an accident on the way to the hospital lab, be sure to have the police rush the sample to the hospital for you. Tell them to flash the lights and use the siren." He had us rolling with laughter.

Then he looked at me and said, "I'm going to schedule you for a diagnostic laparoscopy to check for endometriosis, which I suspect is the primary cause of your infertility."

"Endometriosis? I asked a doctor if I could have that and he said no."

"I believe he was wrong. The symptoms we have discussed are classic. Had you been coming to me years ago I would have looked at that first. Are you familiar at all with the disease?"

"A little, on the way to Washington D.C. earlier this month, Horace and I stopped at a discount bookstore and found a book on endometriosis."

"Endometriosis is a disease that affects nearly ten percent of women, many of whom don't even know they have it. A lot of women with the disease also have fertility problems. Endometrial tissue, normally found only inside the uterus grows outside it and attaches to other organs and forms scar tissue, which can deform the internal organs if it gets too severe. It can also cause distortion of the anatomy, and/or hormonal abnormalities. No one really knows why it happens, but we know that it usually tends to run in families. Now the laparoscopy is a minor surgical procedure, and depending on what we find, I may be able to remove the scar tissue right then. If not, we may have to schedule an operation."

"How much experience do you have with this procedure?" I asked.

"I was one of the first doctors in Ohio to use the laparoscope. It's a simple procedure, usually lasting no more than 30 minutes. We make two incisions, one in your navel, and the other just slightly above it. After it's over, you won't even know you had anything done. I've been using the laparoscope pretty much since it first came out and I am the best."

We both liked his confidence. He wasn't boastful or arrogant, simply self-assured. That's what we were looking for, someone confident in their healing abilities.

"Since I've been doing it, I have only rarely had to actually do a laparotomy to remove endometrial tissue, most of the time I am able to remove any scar tissue I find with a laparoscope. If I do have to operate, it's only because you have too much scar tissue to effectively or safely remove via the laparoscope. Don't worry; you can still wear a bikini afterwards." He laughed.

"Seriously, I will not do a surgery unless it is absolutely necessary, and I wouldn't do anything you didn't want me to do." I liked this man!

My laparoscopy was scheduled for July 27th.

I had to be at the hospital around 6 AM even though the procedure wouldn't take place until 11 AM. It was pretty weird going through it all because I have never been in the hospital for anything other than broken bones or cuts; even though this was an outpatient procedure it was serious business.

One minute I'm in the surgery room getting anesthesia and counting to 100 (I only got to five), and the next thing I know I'm waking up with your daddy and mom standing over me.

"Doc said you did well, although it turned out that you had so much scar tissue that he had to stop the procedure. You have Stage IV endometriosis and you have probably had it since you were fifteen."

"And I always thought you were skipping school because you were embarrassed about being on your cycle." Mom said.

"Um, mom, they wouldn't know unless I told them." I said groggily.

"I didn't know. Remember you used to be so embarrassed to buy the pads that you'd send Jimmy to do it?"

"That's true, but you know I loved school and never missed unless I was really sick. Okay, except for the few times I deliberately skipped classes."

"When did you skip classes?"

"Oooh, I'm sleepy." I said, pretending to fall back asleep.

"Anyway," Your daddy interrupted. "Doc said you're going to have to have a laparotomy. It's major abdominal surgery, but once he removes all the lesions you should have no problem conceiving. But it is major surgery, and you will be in the hospital for at least three to five days. The surgery is more invasive than the laparoscopy. You're going to have a scar of about six inches."

"A six inch scar?"

"Yes, but you won't really see it, because it will be a bikini cut."

"Oh, okay."

"There are some risks too." He said.

"Like what?" I asked still lightheaded.

"Like the formation of new adhesions, infection," he hesitated, "death."

But that's a minor risk; they have to tell you that though. Plus you will be off work at least six weeks and it will be months before your body fully recovers."

"So what happens now?"

"Well he's scheduled an appointment for you to see him, and he'll schedule the surgery then. So for now, you heal up from this, then we move forward."

"I am so excited to finally have some answers." Mom said.

A few weeks later we met with Dr. Watson at his office and afterwards I had a better understanding of why the surgery was necessary. At the surgical consultation, he showed us photos from the laparoscopy. The scar tissue was so bad that it had literally glued my ovaries to my uterus, pulling them out of alignment from the fallopian tubes.

"The good news is that Horace can get you pregnant; he just hasn't had any hills to conquer, but he will soon." He said smiling. "The surgery is scheduled for September 21, and you can start trying to conceive eight weeks afterwards."

We are so excited! I thank God that the endometriosis was not discovered when I was in high school because if it had it been discovered earlier, doctors might have suggested a hysterectomy. That's what happened to my neighbor, and countless other women. My cramps were so bad back then who knows what I might have permitted.

"Lord we would not have chosen this path, yet it must be the best path for us because you placed us on it. What an awesome task it must be to direct the lives of two people— now one. What a symphony we must be? What a beautiful, harmonic, melodic arrangement? What heart stopping music you must be making. Lord, I look forward to seeing Your symphony complete!"

Love Mommy

> *"Unless Your law had been my delight,*
> *I would then have perished in my affliction."*—Psalm 119:92

September 28, 2000

Dear Children:

One week ago at 7:45 AM I was being cut open. I'm telling you, you doggone sure better appreciate this some day! This is such an invasive procedure but I did it because I believe it is what I must do to get to you.

> ... *in faithfulness You have afflicted me. Let... Your merciful kindness be my comfort...Let Your tender mercies come to me, that I may live...Unless Your law had been my delight, I would then have perished in my affliction. I will never forget Your precepts, for by them You have given me life....*
> **Psalm 119:65-96**

At the hospital things seemed so surreal. So many people prayed for us, and their prayers brought me a peace throughout the whole ordeal. The night before we sat on the edge of the bed held hands and prayed too.

That morning Mom and Mrs. Arnold beat us to the hospital. After I changed from my clothes into the hospital gown, we exchanged small talk as she took my vitals and gave me instructions on what to do and what was going to happen. Then I lay down on the cot, asking her to please let Doctor Watson know I wanted to see him before he got started. The night before the operation a tornado was in the Xenia/Yellow Springs area and I was concerned that he wouldn't make it to the hospital.

She promised to do so, and then placed the I.V. in my arm. Then she let my family in to see me.
    "Are you nervous?" Your daddy asked.
    "No, surprisingly I am not. I don't understand why, but I am at

peace. In some small way I think I know how mom must have felt when she had her surgeries. One way or another I am now in God's hands."

It's funny the things you think about during moments like those, things that remind you to trust the Lord you know. Like when your Uncle Jimmy accidentally slammed the front door on my finger, shattering all the bones in it. As the doctor was repairing my finger he told me that I would never re-grow a fingernail due to the severity of the damage. I confidently looked up at him and said, "Yes I will!" And I did.

I don't know where that kind of faith came from. Don't misunderstand me; God is not obligated to heal us. He is not a genie in a bottle we can rub to get our way. Yet, we have to know in our hearts that He is powerful enough to heal us should He desire to do so and we have to know the promises He has made to us.

Abraham would not have offered up his son if He weren't fully persuaded that God could and would raise him up from the dead? NO WAY! But Abraham knew the promises of God *for him* and that in Isaac they would be fulfilled. Abraham had such a relationship with God that he knew God could not lie! This God said that he would become a father of many nations. He understood that God is the giver of life.

And David, do you really think he would've stood up to Goliath if he didn't know his God? Like Abraham David had such a relationship with his God that he KNEW his God could not lie! God had said David would be king over Israel. That couldn't happen if David was dead. He knew he could defeat Goliath because he trusted in the one who made the promise.

I trust in this same powerful and mighty God, but I also understand that He is Sovereign. Phillip Yancey in his book, *Where is God When it Hurts*, helps us to understand those times when God doesn't seem to resolve our suffering as we desire. Not only does he provide a Biblical perspective on pain and its purpose, but he also helps us to recognize that trials and afflictions are often designed to help us develop a closer relationship with God.

During the ordeal we wonder why? I would never have chosen this path for myself. It is a path that causes too much pain. It's too difficult, too hard. But when it's over we thank God for the tests and for the storms because they bring us closer to Him. That's the power! That's God! That's His peace.

But what does it really require to see the fulfillment of the promise? It requires *faith*, *testimony*, and *proof*.

FAITH

> *"Give ear to my words, O LORD, consider my meditation. Give heed to the voice of my cry...I will direct it to You and I will look up."*
> **Psalm 5:1-3**

We must have confidence in the creator of the universe and we must know His promises, **and which promises apply to us.**

God told Adam and Eve (who at that time represented all of mankind) to be fruitful and multiply. This was the command God gave to the inhabitants of the world, of which I am one. In searching the scriptures I found that *through God's grace and divine plan* everyone that had a difficult time conceiving eventually did after much prayer and sometimes much heartache. It didn't always happen right away, but in due course of time it eventually happened.

TESTIMONY

> *"Glory in His holy name; let the hearts of those rejoice who seek the LORD!"*
> **Psalm 105:3**

After we have faith or believe, what do we do with that assurance? The saints of the last days overcame by the word of their testimony. God who created heaven and earth will hear my voice, and regardless of *how* and *when*, and *if* He chooses to answer my prayer I can still confidently affirm that He cares for me, knows me by name, and I am important in His sight.

PROOF

"For as the heaven is high above the earth, so great is His mercy toward them that fear Him."
Psalm 103:11

Faith is the substance (matter, confidence) of things hoped for, the EVIDENCE of things unseen. Everyday, humans do things to prove their faith in people, things. We get in our cars and drive because we have faith that our vehicle will get us safely to our destination.

We faithfully take our prescriptions because we are persuaded that they will bring the relief we need. Why then is it such a hard thing for us to trust that God has our lives in His hands?

David sat in those lonely fields crafting his weapon of choice-a slingshot. He practiced with it, and he took time to choose just the right stones for use. If he did not trust in himself, his weapon, his God, he would not have taken the time out to create it, select choice stones, and practice. He knew doing so could one day mean the difference between life and death. You see where I'm going. This journal is my weapon, the words are the stones, and the act of writing is my practice. Through them I will conquer this enemy of infertility and overcome the sadness, depression and despair.

But I digress.

Dr. Watson arrived at 7:30 AM, and the nurse sent him to see me. Content that he was okay and that no other doctor had been called to operate on me, I lie back down and let the Valium I'd been given work its magic. Everyone kisses me and they whisk me away.

All I remember from that point on is being lifted from the gurney to the table and being given oxygen. Once again it was lights out for me!

I awoke surprised to find that I wasn't in pain. Dr. Watson was using an experimental *"pain pouch"* inserted in the incision. I barely had any pain the whole time I was in the hospital or since I've been home. The only time I wanted to cry was when were transferring me from recovery to my room. They laid me on my side and I wanted them to lay me on my back, but they said they had to lay me that way for a few hours because the anesthesia could cause me to vomit and I might choke on it.

When daddy, mom and Mrs. Arnold came in they asked how I was doing.
"I was okay until they put me on my side and it hurts terribly."
"I'm just surprised you are not still out of it," said Mrs. Arnold.
"Me too," said Mom.
"Well, this post surgical gas is awful. Man it feels terrible. It's like it's all up in there, but won't come out."
"So, did they tell you anything," asked daddy.
"Just that I cannot eat until I pass gas. I don't know how they think I am going to make it without food."
"I'm not talking about that." He laughed. "I mean did they tell you anything about the surgery?"
"Oh. Nope."
"Dr. Watson said you also almost got fried. You left your hairpins in."
"Oh man, I forgot! What exactly could have happened?"
"I don't know, I guess with all the electrical stuff in there you could've gotten shocked. I don't know that it would've killed you or anything, but I'm sure it wouldn't have felt good."
"I guess my hair would've gotten fried then. That would've been funny. Remember when my phony pony fell off when I had that test a few years ago?" I said to mom.
"Yeah, that was hilarious. I thought that woman was going to have a heart attack. She thought she made your hair fall out!" We all cracked up.

"Dr. Watson came out all happy and told us that everything went well." Your daddy interjected. "It took a little longer because there was so much scar tissue, but he removed it, as well as removed cysts that were on both ovaries. He also re-checked your tubes for blockage and they were clear. He also mentioned something about fixing you up. I'm not sure what that means but he said it the way a mechanic does when he's finished giving a car a tune up."

"He also mentioned something about temporarily suspending your uterus to help you heal." Mom said.

"Suspended my uterus, with what?" I freaked out because I had this vision of metal tubes sticking out of my stomach.

"With dissolvable sutures, he said."

"Oh. Okay." I pretended to understand.

"Dr. Watson seemed surprised that I wasn't running around the room yelling 'heehaw!'"

When you have faith you already see the fulfillment of the dream.
You've already lived that moment so when it finally comes, you are peacefully speechless. You have already said to God and to the world what needed to be said, so you are grateful—***beyond words***.

> *"We shall not mount up very high if we only surrender trust in theory, or in our especially religious moments…We must meet our disappointments, our thwartings, our persecutions, our malicious enemies, our provoking friends, our trials, our temptations of every sort, with an active, experimental attitude of surrender and trust."*—**Hannah Whitehall Smith**

This is all too real for me as I allow God to fight this battle against infertility caused by advanced endometriosis. It's very easy to tell others to trust God, but when it comes to my own trust, well then, that's another story. I know that God is able, but I struggle because I am often unsure that He is willing. But now I can no longer trust in theory, but in that person who is my Father, my Savior, my Comforter, and my Guide.

Love Mommy

*"Can a woman forget her sucking child...yea, they may forget, yet I will not forget thee...I have graven thee upon the palms of my hands...—**Isaiah 49:15, 16***

October 3, 2000

Dear Children:

I came downstairs on the day of mom's birthday for the second time since my operation. I wasn't supposed to, but Janet brought dinner and no one was here to lock the door behind her. I didn't want to do too much, but I thought if mom could be strong through her surgeries, why shouldn't I. You never think about how much you take your health for granted until you are not even able to do the simplest things.

Your dad's been taking care of all the chores and housework, and needed to run some errands, before leaving he asked what I was doing for the day.

"I don't know. It's not like there's a whole lot I can do."

"You need to go outside and enjoy the sun for a while."

"I don't want to go outside. I already went downstairs once today and I don't want to overdo it."

"You're fine. You can handle it. I'll even help you."

"But I'm in pain, and unless you plan on carrying me downstairs, I can't handle it." I cried in pretend agony.

"Stop being so melodramatic, we both know you're not in that much pain!"

"I'll just sit upstairs in this here chair, thank you very much."

"You're going downstairs. If your mother can handle it, so can you. So get moving."

"How rude!" Nevertheless around 11 AM I turned off the TV, washed up, slowly made my way downstairs and fixed myself a cup of coffee. I checked the voice mail, returned a few calls, drank some coffee and ate some grapes.

By then your daddy had returned and I was outside sitting on the patio writing. I was having a good time until some stupid bee crawled under my blanket and stung me on the leg. My body was already feeling all swollen and weird, and now this!

"Ahhhh!" I cried, knowing your dad couldn't hear me all the way upstairs. I removed the covers and examined my leg. "Oh shoot, Oh shoot." I said making a move that caused pain to course through my abdomen. Now I had pain in my leg, stomach, and back. I tried to call your dad, and when he didn't respond I slowly got out of the chair and made my way to the patio door. Your dad had opened it for me so I could get in the house faster if I needed to rather than going through the back door, so you can imagine my surprise when I went to open it and found it was LOCKED! I banged on the door. "Why did he lock the door?" I asked the imaginary person standing next to me. Receiving no response, I staggered to the back door on the side of the house, and managed to get it open at the exact moment your dad appeared.

"What's wrong?"

"I got stung by a bee." Before I know it I am crying a Mississippi River of tears.

"Baby, it's okay."

"No it's not, because I don't even know why I'm crying. It's just a bee sting. I didn't cry through mom's surgeries, or my own, and here I am huffing and snuffling over a bee sting."

"Maybe that's the problem."

"What do you mean?" I said through my tears.

"C'mon Lena, all the pressure over the last year had to come out eventually. It might seem weird, but your pressure valve finally exploded. You just had all you could take. Now come on upstairs so I can get the stinger out and clean it." I followed him upstairs complaining about the pain the whole time.

"It feels like someone is stabbing me in my leg with a knife."

"You'll be alright."

Later that day I had a follow-up appointment with Dr Watson. He entered the room with his classic smile and asked how we were doing.

"Why are you still wearing the abdominal brace?"

"I thought I was supposed to wear it until you said to take it off."

"You only needed it for a few days after the surgery." He laughed

"Hey, I didn't know." I laughed back.

"Let me check your abdomen." He pulled back the steri-strips and beamed with pride as he examined the results of his work. "Cool, the scar is barely visible. Doesn't that look good?" he asked your dad.

"Wow!" he exclaimed.

I couldn't see anything over my swollen belly, so I just had to take their word for it.

"You're ready to drive now," he said as he finished.

"I don't think so."

"Oh, yeah," your dad said.

"Oh no," I said.

"Oh yeah," Dr. Watson said. "You're ready to roll."

"But what about the excruciating pain I had when my cycle started in the middle of the night?

"That's because your uterus is suspended to help the healing process. It should be fully dropped by your next cycle so you shouldn't have any pain."

"What about the numbness in my leg?"

"The bikini cut, is an incision across more nerves than the traditional, more invasive abdominal cut. As the nerves heal, your legs will return to normal."

"What about sex?" Of course your daddy asked that question.

"Whenever she's ready and you can start trying to have kids in a month, but until then, use condoms. Don't wait too long you gotta start on those twins. Or maybe triplets! I'm about due for some triplets."

"I don't think so, Dr. Watson, though a couple of years ago my mom dreamed that Horace was getting out of the car with two little boys who looked just like him. That would be one way of making up for lost time."

"Well, stranger things have happened. I've already talked to my friends about you in case after six months you are still not pregnant."

"Oh yeah," your dad asked.

"You're going to get those triplets one way or another, huh?" I said.

William Harding declared that God has prepared a Mercy seat, a Throne of grace to sit on; that we may come to God and He may hear us and receive us. There we can bring our petitions to God.

Love Mommy

*"Be kindly affectionate one to another with brotherly love;
in honor preferring one another."*
Romans 12:10

October 14, 2000

Dear Children:

"Okay doctor; give it to me straight, can you help me?" Mom asked bravely.

"Well, let me tell you what's going on, then I'll tell you if I can help you." Then using a diagram of the digestive system, and a pad to draw pictures, he said. "The colonoscopy you took last Friday revealed the presence of three more tumors in your colon. One is located in the ascending colon, one in the transverse, and one in the descending." He continued. "The good news is that for some reason your tumors tend to grow in lumps, as opposed to most cancers which grow along a flat plane and spread out. This is the only reason you have survived for as long as you have. Your type of cancer is easier to remove. The bad news is your going to have to have another surgery. We're going to have to remove your large intestine."

All things considered, we both took the news pretty well, though I'm not sure if either of us really understood what his words really meant.

"So, what does that mean doctor?" I finally asked.

"Well, to tell the truth, we never expected your mom to live this long. We consider her a miracle."

"That's because I told her she's not allowed to go anywhere until after my children are born."

"I told you I'm going to be in the Bahamas when you get pregnant. You're not driving me crazy." Mom said smiling.

"So, if you remove her large intestine, how will she live? I mean..." I couldn't contemplate the enormity of it all, nor consider what he was saying.

"Well, you can live without your large intestine. You just can't live without your small one."

"Really, that's incredulous!" I exclaimed.

"I guess I'm going to have another colostomy." She said dejectedly.

"No, not this time," he said.

"I won't?" She said happily, "How is that possible?"

"We're not going to remove it entirely. You'll still have a little bit left. You'll just go more often because there won't be much to hold anything in."

I wondered why he didn't do that in the first place. Perhaps if he had we wouldn't be here now. I wanted to ask, but I didn't.

"So, is she going to be alright? I mean I don't want her going through another surgery if..." Again, I couldn't say what I was thinking.

"Again, I'll be honest with you, no one expected your mom to last this long. I mean she's had four surgeries in the last two years."

Since he felt good, we did too. Finally, there seemed to be some light at the end of the tunnel. Still I could not shake that dream. I know God is with her; yet still I can't help but wonder what the end will be.

The next day I took mom to her family doctor for a consultation.
She sings, quotes scripture, and preaches while we wait. I'm not sure if she's talking to me or to herself in general. Paul and Silas in jail and the earth shook, interspersed with her singing. I know this must be even harder for her since it hasn't been that long since her own mom died.

Sometimes it's difficult to know what she is really thinking. Despite her small frame she is a really strong woman both emotionally and physically. She doesn't like to complain. So it's hard to know where her head is, but I guess you've got to go through some things to understand.

It's like you start out praying about your situation, you know sad and all, then God gives you a taste of His mercy and grace on your life and then you're shouting for joy. I was ruminating on it later that day as I pulled weeds from the flower garden, when my neighbor broke my thoughts.

"So, how have you been?"

"Didn't I tell I had to have surgery?"

"No! Surgery, do you mind if I ask you why?"

"Not at all, I had stage IV endometriosis."

"Oh yeah, I know what you are talking about. I had a hysterectomy in 1978 because of endometriosis."

"Oh man, I never knew that."

"Yeah, back then that was pretty much the answer. Is everything alright?"

"Yeah, we should be able to have kids pretty soon."

It's late in life, but Moses was older than me when he led the children of Israel out of Egypt.

"Lord, let us have that strength, but not only us, give strength to all those waiting to birth the dreams you placed in them."

Love Mommy

"For it was fitting for Him, for whom are all things and by whom are all things, in bringing many sons to glory, to make the captain of their salvation perfect through suffering."
Hebrews 2:10

October 22, 2000

Dear Children:

Mom and I had prayer while she was in the prep area for her most recent surgery. Your daddy then came in and your grandma asked him to pray.
 "What, you don't trust my prayers," I teased. Then we kissed and hugged her.

Seven hours later the surgeon came out.
 "I apologize for keeping you waiting. The operation took much longer than we expected and I hate to say this but it did not go well." Using handmade drawings to illustrate his point he continued, "I was very optimistic that your mom would survive, and things were going really well. We had removed her colon and had attached the small intestine to what was left of her large intestine and we were just about to close when I had a thought to look underneath her small intestine. When I saw it, it just tore my heart out. I hate this disease. Under her small intestine was cancer everywhere. The CAT scan did not pick it up, but it was all over, and it cannot be removed."
 "What do you mean it cannot be removed?" Staci asked, while the rest of us looked on speechless.
 "It's too much, and too much is attached to vital organs. Major blood vessels are running through them, and if we removed it, it would kill her instantly."
 "How much time does she have left?" I asked hesitantly.
 "If she survives, she'll be in the hospital for a month. After that, she won't live more than six months. Sadly, I don't think she's going to leave this hospital."

I never knew what the statement "*it hit me like a ton of bricks*," meant until that moment. That's how I felt, like someone had slammed me into a brick wall, and then dumped another ton of bricks on my head. We were all totally stunned. None of us were prepared for this news. For the first time since mom was diagnosed and started having surgeries I cried. Before there was always a ray of hope, but this time, barring a miracle from heaven, mom was not going to live.

I tell you though she is something else, this morning she was on the phone praying with one of her friends and she was so loud that I had to keep reminding her that she was in a hospital.

"Mom, there are other sick people here, who might not want to be disturbed." I whispered.

"They need prayer too."

"Whoever that is tell them they are not allowed to call back." I teased.

"You hear that?" She said. "We just gonna keep on praising him!"

She wouldn't listen to me and you know what, I decided that she shouldn't. After what she'd been through as far as I was concerned she could do whatever she wanted!

Everyone keeps saying something good must be getting ready to happen soon; something big —something really awesome, special! I question this notion that all this suffering must precede it. Isn't God capable of making that something special come without my mom dying?

Despite it all Mom, has never wavered in her belief of the God of Abraham, Isaac, and Jacob, not even in her darkest hour. No matter what happens, keep believing and trusting in the God of your grandmother.

We are forced to acknowledge that God is the author of not only our salvation but also of our lives. Jesus was made perfect through suffering and as His followers we are often made perfect in the same way. It is our suffering, not our joy that brings us closer to God. T.C. Horton and Charles Hurlburt put it this way, *"The mode and method of perfection is manifested by our Leader. He was tempted; so are we. He* suffered; so must we. He was persecuted; so must we be. The climax for Him and us is glory."

I wish there was some other way, and yet there isn't. If we are to truly know God, then we must know that everything—even our body belongs to Him. It is not that we won't go through trials and tribulations; rather it is *how* we go through them that makes the difference.

"Peace I leave with you, My peace I give to you; not as the world gives do I give to you. Let not your heart be troubled, neither let it be afraid."
John 14:27

"Sudden changes often remind me of my inner self. My emotions...— changing directions with the slightest breeze. There are times when clouds of negativism hang over me; their constant dripping cause dreariness of soul and spirit...I used to be upset, even ashamed of these changing emotions. I thought that a deeply spiritual person should not and would not have these fluctuations of mood."
Gigi Graham Tchividjian.

I thank God for the author of this excerpt, and for the Biblical examples of Gods people who like us experienced emotional ups and downs. These words remind me that while I am passionate, moody, and scared, I am also totally dependent upon God. And God promises us a place that lasts.

Love Mommy

> *"If a man therefore purges himself from these, he shall be a vessel unto honor, sanctified and meet for the master's use, and prepared unto every good work."*—II Timothy 2:21

November 23, 2000

Dear Children:

"She made you come again huh?" Dr. Watson teased daddy.

"I make him come so he can see what women go through."

"You're funny," he said. "When is your next period due?"

"Tomorrow," I responded.

"Do you feel like it's going to come?"

"I think so," I said, disappointed.

"Well, maybe it won't." He said. "How were your last two cycles?"

"Bad."

"Debilitating?" He questioned.

"No a lot like most of them, but from my studies, I expected the first few cycles to be that way."

"Let's take a look at you." He said as he helped me lay down. "I'm telling you when you do get pregnant you're going to have twins, maybe girls."

"Girls, oh no," your dad exclaimed!

"Girls are fun man, you'll love them."

"It's not that, I just don't want to have to kill anybody!"

They are joking and I'm on the table with a hand up my vagina. Couldn't they table this conversation for now?

"So, have you been experiencing any other problems?"

"My ovaries have been hurting and so have my breasts."

"Is the breast soreness in relation to your normal cycle?"

"I think so, except sometimes they hurt at off times. Now that I think of it my PMS symptoms have been askew —off so to speak."

"What do you mean?"

"Like symptoms that would normally occur a few days before my period are now occurring up to two weeks before my cycle starts. The good part is that my PMS is nowhere near as bad as it was before."

"A lot of this is normal." He says washing his hands while talking. "But if after one or two more cycles you're still having severe cramps, call the office." Then he turns back and looks at me with this big grin.

"You must be pleased with your work." I rag.

"Well you look good. Everything feels fine, everything's clean."

"You can tell all that just by feeling?" I asked.

"Sure can."

"You must really be pleased because you have that same look on your face that Horace has on his after he's finished working on one of his cars."

"We'll I am good." He laughed, don't be surprised if it doesn't come, but if you are not pregnant in six months I've got my guys on standby for In-Vitro."

"This is going to work. I could never handle poking a needle in my stomach. So thanks for your friends, but we are not going to need them."

I said the words, but I am not sure I really believed them.

This is the first time in my life that I actually could get pregnant and yet I am not expecting it to happen. I don't really know what to feel. Your dad says he is not concerned about what other people say, and I know he means well, but all of him is working properly. Everybody knows that *I'm* the one with the screwed up plumbing!

And what if I do get pregnant, will I have miscarriages over and over again? What if I end up with a tubal pregnancy? What if it's stillborn or has a birth defect? What if I wind up with twins, triplets, quads, etc…? What will I do then? Now I have a whole new set of fears! I never really had to consider all these scenarios before.

"Stop," I tell myself. I must take one step at a time, one day at a time. Right now I would do well to remember Psalm 102 and call out to God in this troubled time. He hears and at the appointed time He favors His children and gives them an inheritance who will praise His name.

"Lord You have brought us this far. I pray I will not be afraid of the future, wondering if You will abandon me there."

Love Mommy

"The walls may look high, as immovable as ever; and prudence may say it is not safe to shout until the victory is actually won. But the faith that can shout in the midst of the sorest stress of temptation, 'Jesus saves me… now!' Such a faith will be sure to win a glorious and speedy victory."
Hannah Whitehall Smith

November 24, 2000

Dear Children:

Sometimes I think I am so numb and empty that I can't feel anymore, and then suddenly I break down crying. I know God didn't play a joke on me, but I still feel like there's an invisible hand slapping me in my face.

It's Thanksgiving Day and all around the country families are gathering with their children; playing with them, chasing them, feeding them. And what do I do–I help them. I'm the faithful assistant who asks, '*Is it okay if Little Mark has a Popsicle? Would Ivory like more turkey?*' I'm the living toy when Kayla or James asks, '*Aunt Marie will you play a game with us?*' I'm the beggar constantly asking; '*Can auntie have a hug?*'"

I love my nieces and nephews, but when the night is over they go home and are tucked in by their parents and all we're left with is our dreams. That and family asking, "So when are you guys going to have some kids of your own?" Why do they care and who gave them the right to ask?

Aw, that's just the way of the world Lena, quit tripping! People are supposed to procreate and when they don't people feel it is their God given right to know why you aren't. I just want to scream, "Well for the record world, it's none of your business!"

"This is impossible!" I yell to no one in particular. "I'm trying to see

You Lord, but it's getting harder and harder. I'm trying to declare Your truth to the world, but You are making it very difficult! How can I deal with all of this? I have lost three jobs in the past three years, mom's dying of Cancer and I'm infertile!

I know You said You would not put more on us than we can bear, but I am not this strong. I can't take this weight anymore. Happy Thanksgiving — yeah right! In the face of all this pain I try to convince myself that I am thankful for hope, but how can I truly be thankful for something I am on the verge of losing?"

> *"Get a clear view of Him who can deal with the impossibility of your life...The path of the child of God from the wilderness to Canaan is by way of facing the impossible and looking up to a risen Christ and getting hold of Him."*—**Alan Redpath**

"I'm trying Lord, I really am."

Love Mommy

> *"Then we who are alive and remain shall be caught up together with them in the clouds to meet the Lord in the air. And thus we shall always be with the Lord.*
> ***I Thessalonians 4:17, 18***

December 18, 2000

Dear Children:

"They came to the house and told my mom they thought I might have syphilis." Mom said. "I'm not sure if it was the state government officials or Federal, since I was only seven years old. *They* said they needed to take me away so they could check me out. I don't know why me of all people, but mom, being ignorant on the disease thought, 'Oh my God, yes take her, do whatever you have to do to make it all right.' She didn't know that it was impossible for me to have had syphilis. That's why I didn't want that epidural, because they were doing spinal taps on me when I was there."

"Spinal taps! Oh my God they were experimenting on you! It's almost like the Tuskegee experiment. They've probably been watching you all these years. Maybe that's why you have cancer." I said, while the movie *Conspiracy Theory* played in my head.

God knows I hate that mom is sick, but it's because of the sickness that I have learned so much more about her.

"Everybody there was black and I was the youngest person so the older girls treated me like I was a baby doll. They combed my hair, played with me and read to me. It was fun. I wasn't old enough to really realize what was going on, or that my mom was in anguish for an entire week waiting for word and for me to come home. They wouldn't let anyone come visit me; and when they brought me back home all they said to mom was, 'She's fine.' I went looking for that building when I got older and it was gone. Before I could ask more questions, she was on to something else.

"My daddy didn't want me to get married? I'm not really sure why. Maybe he just wasn't ready for his little girl to get married.

Anyway, on the day of my wedding, he decides that he needs to go visit one of the church deacons who'd been arrested for running moonshine."

"Moonshine, what's the deacon doing running moonshine?"

"I don't know but he made me mad because daddy didn't make it back in time and I was so devastated that I cried like a baby. Everyone tried to calm me down. Mr. Ramey ended up having to give me away."

"Mr. Pinchey Butt?"

"Yes," She said laughing. "It was terrible."

When mom was in college she lived with a well to do black family and helped run the house. Mr. Ramey used to sneak pinches on her butt, until one day mom hit him in the balls and that was the last of that.

"That's how I ended up having a Catholic wedding." She continued. Catholics had the money and the society life. The whole town turned out for that wedding, everybody but my daddy."

"The whole town!" I asked incredulous. "But in the pictures all I've ever seen were a few people. I'd always thought you had a small intimate wedding."

"Are you kidding, the whole town came, including some of the boys who used to like me. I guess they wanted to see who got me."

"Shortly after our wedding your dad got stationed in Japan. He wanted me to come with him right away, but I wanted to stay in school, after a year one of my professors told me that he was once in a similar situation and wanted his wife to come with him and she wouldn't. I knew my professor was gay, so I figured I'd better go to Japan because I didn't want to be responsible for turning your daddy gay."

"Mom, I seriously don't think that would've made him gay." I doubled over with laughter. "If anything you should've been worried about those Japanese whore houses."

"I didn't even think about those!"

So in 1963, fearing her husband might become a homosexual, this 20-year-old country girl, who'd only been as far as St. Louis, embarked on an exciting journey to Japan. Mom was like a celebrity; a black woman going to Japan!

"Your dad booked me on the S.S. Orsova and I applied for my Visa and went through the entire shots process. It just so happened that around that time some friends of mine were driving to Omaha, Nebraska to visit their son. I rode with them and caught the bus from Omaha to San Francisco where my ship was scheduled to depart.
Once I got on the bus in Omaha I realized that for the first time I could sit wherever I wanted! I wasn't automatically relegated to the back of the bus, and no one looked at me funny when I sat in the front next to a white person. I'd never done that before! You'd think I'd be scared, but I knew the Lord was with me."

"I think I would have been."

"I think I was too excited to be scared. The bus trip was nice and extremely scenic. And when we went through Wyoming, I saw real Indians, well I mean Native Americans, for the first time in my life! One of our stopovers was in Reno, Nevada. I saw slot machines!"

She said it like a little child seeing Disney World for the first time.

"After we left Salt Lake City around midnight, our bus got a flat tire in what seemed like the middle of the desert. When we finally got to San Francisco I spent the night with Lawrence's mom, your Aunt Mary belle's ex-husband. We rode the trolley cars and went to a nightclub."

"You at a nightclub, I just can't see that!"

"Yes me." She said. "Finally the time came for me to board the ship and it was huge, the largest passenger ship on the P& O Orient Lines. It was full of workers, people of all nationalities I never thought I'd meet. And the food was great. My cabin mates were all mostly Japanese and everyone was extremely nice. My roommates were Hatsuko..."

"That's who you almost named me after right." I interrupted.

"Yes, and there was Yakuso, and another older lady whose name I can't recall. Two of them spoke English and we had a blast. "At dinner I was allowed to sit with people of different races. Here I was this little girl from the backwoods of Mississippi, never having any experiences with anyone other than black people, and I am hanging out and having a good time with white people, Hispanic people, and Japanese people! Who would have thought? It was like I was in a dream. I'd never been with anyone outside my own race before, not even in college. I mean for goodness sake the entire town I grew up in was black, so this was something else."

"That is, uh, was something else. Wow."

"We lived on that ship for thirteen days like a little family. They used to tease me because I had a favorite alcoholic drink called a Pimm."

"You were drinking alcohol?"

"Hey, what can I say?" She laughed weakly. "I didn't order much because I didn't have much money. Everyone knew I was on my way to meet my husband so they looked after me and gave me a good farewell celebration before I left."

"That was nice of them."

"It was wasn't it? At one point we had a layover in Los Angeles and I went out on the town with Hatsuko. She was Episcopalian and had host groups to meet her at both the layovers in Los Angeles and Hawaii."

"You weren't scared? I mean, what if something happened?"

"I should have been scared; we went to a Spanish restaurant where women danced on tables. I'd never seen Mexican people before. I remember them doing the *Mexican Hat Dance*. It was an educational experience like out of nowhere!" She smiled at the memories. "While I was there we visited the San Gabriel Mission and hung out at Disneyland.

"In Hawaii, we visited a pineapple plantation, the national cemetery and Pearl Harbor. I saw a ship that still had oil all over it. We also had dinner with a Hawaiian family. I was eating well until they told me I was eating clams, which I spit out in my napkin. I'm sure they all had a good laugh on me."

"I'm blown away."

"When I finally got to Japan, we landed in Yokohama, where I was held by the Japanese Immigration Authorities because they thought I was a spy. I don't know why they would think I was a spy, or what was wrong with my Visa, except that I thought my picture was ugly. They took me to a small room where they interrogated me. They asked me all kinds of questions like where I went to school. When I answered them, they said they never heard of Mississippi Valley State College or Etta Bena, Mississippi."

"They were probably just fascinated with you and used that as an excuse to detain you a while longer. You just might possibly have been the first black woman they'd ever seen." I said.

"I don't know, but they finally agreed to let me stay for twenty four hours."

"Do you think they were going to make you go home?"

"I really didn't think so, but your father was so distraught until he was able to work with the military and the American Consulate to straighten things out. I just chalked it up as one more part of the great adventure."

"What happened then?"

"Well they finally worked it out. Your dad was stationed at Fuchu Air Base in Fuchu, Japan. Since he wasn't an officer we had to live in military approved housing within a Japanese neighborhood. In Japan everything was little. We had a little house, with a little dog, and little Japanese friends. We visited little Japanese restaurants in the little hill country with one of his service mates who had a Japanese wife."

"What else did you do while you were there? Did you ever get bored?"

"No, not really, your dad got me a job as a bus monitor for the military brats of the officers. The Japanese women taught me how to catch the train. I rode the bus with the kids to the high school in Tokyo and caught the train back to the base. Later in the day I'd catch the train back to the schools so I could ride back on the bus with the kids."

"How was that? I mean how did the kids treat you considering it was the early '60's and you were black?"

"I never had any problems. They used to talk to me about everything and we'd have a good time."

"Man this is interesting. You should have kept a journal."

"I was there for 11 months before I got pregnant with Jimmy. Then I had to come back home."

Mom started getting tired, but it was fantastic talking to her.

> ***Still…****I rise…Letting my soul flow with the beauty of the sunset*
> *Becoming one, with the fullness of the sky So you see, I didn't really die!*
> *I comprise the rainbow and I comprise the sun*
> *Like the unity In the Fathers kingdom-The Son and I are one*
> *Still I'm rising…Joining new worlds, new realities*
> *Riding each cascading wave, of heaven's celestial seas*

Mom's going to die I know that now and the only comfort, the only consolation I have is that I know where she is going and I know someday I'll be with her again.

Love Mommy

"Jesus is our patience; our power to wait; our power to hope."
Mommy

February 4, 2001

Dear Children:

"Hey girl, we are going to have another baby!" Sharon said excitedly.

"I'm really happy for you two." I told my friend.

"I'm truly grateful to God, sometimes I feel like I don't deserve them considering what I did…"

She didn't have to finish; I knew what she was talking about.

"You understand now that He doesn't hold it against you."

"I know it took me so long to call you because I didn't know how you were going to take it."

"We are always happy to share in the joy of others, so don't ever be afraid to call. Of course I want kids, but I know life's not perfect."

"Wouldn't it really be nice if things really were like we once thought?"

"I spent the weekend at my mom's house looking through old photographs and it made me remember little moments of perfection, you know, things that made me believe in God. Like how the sunlight used to pour in the doors and the windows and I used to sit there basking in its warm glow. Many of those old photos were made into slides and we used to feel like we were movie stars when my Uncle Harry would project them. The images were crisp and clear, and larger than life. It was a little sliver of perfection."

"See, that's why I wasn't going to call you. You're thinking too much."

"Girl, you never have to be afraid to call me." I responded slowly.

"Yes, sometimes it's hard, with these PMS symptoms taunting me, I run to the calendar to see how much closer I am to the due date of my period."

"Why?" She asked.

"I don't know why I do that. It's as if I think I can magically make it stop coming, but none of that means I can't be happy for my friends."

"What if your period doesn't come?" She asked. "Are you going to spend the next nine months worrying about miscarrying, or birth problems?"

"I'll try not to. I'll try to focus on better things."

"Marie, I know you." She calls me by my middle name. "You are the world's greatest hypochondriac, when you get pregnant, try not to worry about all that."

"Lord, tell me which way I should go, for I cannot even take the next step without Your power. This is a battle I cannot fight, a victory I cannot attain apart from Your help. This pain and confusion is driving me towards hopelessness... Just when I thought it couldn't get any worse the stakes were raised.

Nevertheless I will go on, trusting that whatever way You turn me will be the direction ordained for me from before the foundation of the world, and in doing so I regain a sense of power over my malady."

Love Mommy

> "But we all, with unveiled face, beholding as in a mirror the glory of the Lord, are being transformed into the same image from glory to glory, just as by the Spirit of the Lord."
> **II Corinthians 13:8**

June 14, 2001

Dear Children:

Mom has grown worse and I'm working harder than ever. She doesn't eat much, she's lost a lot of weight, she's got these dark circles around her eyes, and she's so skinny it looks like she's been in a concentration camp. Sometimes I see her lying in the bed asleep with her hands folded over her chest. It freaks me out because she looks just like she's lying in a coffin.

The whole time worried that if I'm pregnant I'll miscarry from all the extra stress. I hope she lives long to hear me say I am pregnant. This is my second month on Clomid. If don't conceive this time Dr. Watson is going to send me to a specialist. He's still holding out for twins, and mom is convinced we will have twins too because of her dream.

I can't worry about that though because God is in control and when it's time for you to come, then you will come. It's hard to accept that you might not get here before mom dies. I keep thinking, "God you've got to give me a break sometime, somewhere."

> *It's my reasonable service, For all the things you've done for me*
> *Like when you held me tight, when I skinned my knee*
> *For how you came to every game, That I played in school*
> *Lovin' me despite the times, That I broke your rules*
> *Always there behind the scenes, Believing' in my every dream*
> *So it's my reasonable service, To serve you*

For now, I am her faithful servant, finding a few stolen moments for fun in between caring for her. Aunt Lois is here for a while helping us take care of mom, so later that evening, your daddy and I went for a walk, and then we sat on the porch reminiscing about times we got into trouble as kids.

We laughed so hard that our stomachs hurt. Before bed I checked on mom and she said, "Marie, Lois, I'm going to beat this thing. I want to live so I can help raise my grandbabies."

"You mean you're not going to run off to the Bahamas when I get pregnant?" I teased. Mom used to always say that since I'm such a hypochondriac.

"No, I think I'll stick around." She said. Lois and I simply nodded and smiled. What could we say? Who am I to limit God, am I not believing Him for a miracle myself? What will it take for me to get pregnant? I know God is sovereign, but why not ask; all He can do is say no? I was already prepared for that. But what if He says yes?

"My grace is sufficient for you for my strength is made perfect in weakness..."
II Corinthians 12:9

Still, I thank Him for the peace for what I know in my heart—that through much tribulation she will enter the kingdom of God. Like Charles Finney said, I will rest upon Him and be quiet, lay my heart in His hand, and nestle down in His perfect will, and have no anxiety.

"Father thank You for Your gardens; the one that leads to death, the one that leads to life, and the one we will partake of for eternity. Though life seems hard You allow rain and wind in the garden of our life and these storms help us to become beautiful. I don't like the storms. They make me apprehensive and afraid, but eventually they do draw me nearer to You. In them I see my weaknesses and my frailties and I learn that when I come to the end of me-You are there."

Love Mommy

"For we know that if our earthly house is destroyed, we have a building from God, a house not made with hands, eternal in the heavens."—II Corinthians 5:1

August 31, 2001

Dear Children:

"Many people don't go the way she did. I checked on her and she was breathing, and I came back 20 minutes later as she took her last breath. She just breathed in and that was it. It was really, really peaceful, no struggle, no fear, nothing." Her Hospice nurse said.

She died Thursday, June 21st at 2:20 A.M.

I went downtown today to pick up some papers from the probate court. On the way I walked through the department store where we both once worked. As I passed the perfume counter I thought of mom. We used to go there on Downtown Dayton Days and on holidays to shop. She'd always try whatever perfume she could get her hands on, driving anyone who was with her nuts with all those aromas! It became a game, with her trying to get at as much perfume as she could, and us trying to stop her.

All these memories flooded my head and I finally allowed myself to cry all the tears I wanted to cry, desperately missing my mom and those times we used to share.

Her last coherent words to me were, "You were right to bring me here." I thank her for that. I struggled with so much guilt, even though I knew Hospice was the right place for her.

That night when she fell asleep she never really woke back up, just drifted in and out from there. I prayed the whole day that she would just wake up one more time so I could tell her how much I loved her. I asked God to let me see her smile one more time.

Later that night I had a dream and it was so real that I thought I was awake. Mom was smiling the most beautiful smile, and I knew that in God's way, he had answered my prayer. Her physical body was finished, but her spiritual body would live forever and she was happy. When the phone rang early Thursday morning around 2:40 A.M. my heart was at peace. I knew mom was gone.

I Remember
When she was young and strong
When the life of sweetness
Was in her song
Like a lark on high
Singing long and loud
In the day when her back
Stood strong and proud
I remember my mommy

Charles Colson said, *"History is full of examples of God using for His greatest work those who seem most insignificant in man's eyes…The strong need the weak so they can be close to God's strength."*

Mom's name may never be etched into a stone monument raised up by mortal man, but it is etched in God's Book of Life, as well as in the hearts of all she touched.

"Lord grow in me mom's strength. Grow in me her forgiving nature and forbearing spirit, that I may honor her memory. Let me be the faithful servant who trusted wholly in You no matter what I am going through."

Mom is exalted now. She is seated with Christ in heavenly places and robed in God's eternal tunic of righteousness. I miss her, but in the meantime I will always remember her.

Love Mommy

Behold, the kingdom of God is within you."
Luke 17:21

September 1, 2001

Dear Children:

"I'm telling you the shots are not that bad," that's what Craig my high school buddy said. He and his wife are currently going through In-Vitro fertilization.
"Yeah, you say that, but you're not the one taking them."
"I'm telling you Kim will say the same thing."
"I don't know. I still don't believe you guys, but we'll see."

"Now may the Lord of peace Himself give you peace always in every way. The Lord be with you all."
II Thessalonians 3:16

I can't believe I have to do this. I can't do this. I recalled my conversation with Bonita years earlier. But I was doing it; and as we headed to the clinic we were referred to by Dr. Watson, neither one of us ever imagined that we'd be here.

Dr. Bidwell introduced himself and seemed very pleasant. We made small talk for a few minutes, and then got right down to business.
"I've reviewed your case and before we try In-Vitro, I think there's another option we should try first. There's a process called Intra Uterine Insemination, IUI for short, where we inject the sperm directly into the uterus. Sometimes a woman's cervical mucous is simply inhospitable to the man's sperm, and this process allows us to bypass the cervix all together. It's more cost effective than In-Vitro and constitutes far less time and effort."
"How does the process work exactly?" Your daddy asked.
"We collect a sperm sample from Horace on the day of the retrieval. A catheter is placed through the vagina and cervix, and the sperm is injected directly into the uterus. If all goes well, fertilization

will occur naturally from there.

There's a whole series of things you'll have to go through first. I'm going to schedule you for a Hysterosalpinogram (HSG), in this test; dye is shot through your tubes to see if they are blocked. I see you've had one before, but since your surgery they could have become clogged, so we're going to make sure they are open before we start this course of action.

We'll start everything at the beginning of your next menstrual cycle. Here's how the process will work. On the third day of your cycle we'll perform an ultrasound to measure follicle development. On the fifth day of your cycle you'll start taking Clomid and you'll take it for five days. You'll have the HSG on day 10 and on day 11 we'll do a blood test. On day 14 we'll do another ultrasound to again measure follicle development, and if they are ready, you will take the HCG shot that evening. Within thirty-six hours of taking the shot we'll do the insemination."

"Wow! That's a lot of information to swallow."

"Don't worry. We'll give you a schedule and a video so you can learn how to administer the shot." We talked some more about the process, then left to wait for day one.

By day 14, the day of the shot we had gone through quite a bit. You should have seen us agonizing over the injection. I was so scared that your daddy was going to kill me, that I made him read the instructions and watch the video three times before I would allow him to give me the shot. He finally drew it, and when he couldn't remove a tiny air bubble, I called your aunt Chrystal to make sure it was okay. First she laughed good-naturedly at us, and then she reassured us that everything would be fine as long as we massaged the area afterwards to keep it from getting sore.

"I can't do it. I just can't do it." He was so afraid of hurting me.

It was my fault, I was so freaked out that he got nervous, and now he couldn't do it.

"Just do it." I assured him. "I'll be…ouch, what did you do that for?"

"You said get it over with!"

"Yeah, but you could have at least warned me." I said, rubbing my hip.

"Well how was it?"

"All things considered it wasn't that bad."

"I'm good." He beamed with pride.

Thursday morning we dropped the sample off at the lab, returned home, fed the dog, and ate breakfast, before returning to the office at 10 AM for the insemination. Dr. Bidwell was off, so Dr. Burwinkle performed the procedure, explaining everything along the way. Then he had us identify the tube to verify that the sample was ours. I'm thinking, "Oh great, I'm supposed to identify sperm? How am I supposed to do that?" Suddenly I pictured a sperm lineup and me going, "Yeah, that's them, numbers 25-2 million, 4.5 million-6 million, and 7-10 million, etc."

He must have been reading my mind because he said, "We go to great lengths to make sure we have the right samples. As soon as you drop it off we have you write the name and social security number on your sample. When it's transferred into the tube, we write the same information on it. Then we ask you to again verify that this is indeed the same number on the tube you dropped off this morning." It was his SSN, but I mean, c'mon really!

After "identifying" the sperm, I lay down while the catheter was inserted and the sperm injected. I was then instructed to lay flat until the buzzer sounded, after which I could get dressed. It took less than five minutes. Now all I can do is wait till the blood test to measure my progesterone levels* to see if I'm pregnant.

I definitely feel changes in my body, but they warned me the hormones could mimic pregnancy symptoms and I'm scared that that is all they are.

"Hear me when I call, O God of my righteousness! You have relieved me in my distress; have mercy on me and hear my prayer."
Psalm 4:1

"I don't know if I can go through this again." I told your dad later.

"It's not so much the process, but the real stress is in the waiting and the hoping. The emotional toll is far greater than the physical toll."

"For me it's both. I feel like a circus clown forced to perform even though I don't want to. On top of all that I have to miss work and deal with people asking, 'Where were you yesterday?' Like I'm going to tell them I was at home ejaculating into a cup!"

"Well maybe tomorrow it will all be over. I hope they tell us right away."

"Don't worry girl, it won't be long." Janet said when picking up her kids. I'd watched them so she could run some errands. "C'mon girl, God gives Horace this great job out of the blue, and then you find out that they pay for fertility treatments including In-Vitro. If that ain't God I don't know what is!"

"What about that timing? Before we could take advantage of the benefits, we had to have one year of documented proof of infertility. Just think what if I hadn't gone to the doctor last year when I did."

"That's what I'm talking about. You knew that you might have to go through In-Vitro and you totally trusted God to take care of it and He did in a really big way!"

"That's true. Can you believe they pay for up to three attempts at In-Vitro?"

"I'm telling you girl. I just don't believe God brought you all this way to let you down. Just remember, don't bring them to my house when you can't take it anymore." She laughed.

"I guess it's true, you know what they say about seasons and things. Maybe this is finally my season?"

"True that! I mean think about it, with Horace being in school and your mom being sick, and the financial pressure you were under, you couldn't have dealt with the stress of pregnancy."

"You ain't lying about all that. I just have to get this negative tape out of my head that I don't deserve anything good."

"Here let me knock you upside the head and eject it for you."

"Girl, you better go on!" I laughed.

I thank God for encouraging friends because not only does God send the Holy Spirit to comfort us, but He sends friends who we can touch, and hear, and who touch us.

Love Mommy

*"Make a joyful shout to God, all the earth! Sing out the honor of his name; make His praise glorious. Say to God, 'How awesome are Your works!'—**Psalm 66:2-4***

November 11, 2001

Dear Children:

Another Thanksgiving Day is on the way and again I am not feeling very thankful. I was already depressed because of 9/11. All of America was down because of what happened.

I had to speak at a women's conference a few days afterwards and I wondered how in the world I was going to inspire them when I was so depressed. I mean, I'm the captain of my own a crap filled boat. How was I supposed motivate women to rise-to fly, when I hardly felt like rising or flying myself? I tried though. Here's a little of what I said.

"...Nothing in my life has turned out as I planned. Many of you probably feel the same way as well. You never imagined the series of twist and turns life would take you on, leading you to the place where you now are. Like all little girls I dreamed of having a successful career, marrying a rich handsome man, living in a beautiful mansion, and raising a bunch of beautiful children.

I never envisioned the enemies of happiness-death, despair, and despondency to creep in and bring destruction to my dream. Nowhere in my fantasy did these enemies have a place...

For the first ten years of our marriage my husband and I dealt with the pain of infertility alone, too ashamed to share our secret with anyone. I went to doctor after doctor trying to figure out what was wrong. Finally, in June of 2000 I was diagnosed with stage IV endometriosis, the extent of my disease so severe that my ovaries were stuck to my uterus resulting in the infertility.

I was overjoyed to finally have a reason for my infertility and was even more ecstatic to learn that it could be treated. No longer would I have to feel the pitying eyes of my relatives at each re-union. No longer would I have to endure the clichés and trite words from these would be consolers, but who were in reality in-clandestine, subversive afflicters. Saying things like, 'God just needed another flower in His garden?' Or 'You guys can always adopt.'

No longer would we have to endure the spiritual accusations of church friends saying, 'Sis, you just ain't prayed up enough.' Or, 'You just need to trust God more.' And, 'You sure you don't have some secret sin in your life...'

...I was scheduled for surgery and six months after it I still had not conceived. Ten months and several fertility treatments later, still more of the same. Eleven months after my surgery and two-months after my moms death I underwent an intra-uterine insemination procedure. It is a two-week process that consists of monitoring, oral drugs, and injected drugs to stimulate the ovaries to produce extra eggs. The results were good and everything looked well, yet I still had not conceived.

Now I'd had all of life I could take and I finally broke in a way I didn't even think was ever possible. No matter what I had gone through in life before I never wanted to die-until that moment. The agony was too much to bear. I could never make you feel what I felt inside when I first saw the telltale signs of my cycle starting. I literally wanted to curl up and die. I felt like the psalmist who wrote:

> "I am troubled, I am bowed down greatly; I go mourning all the day long. For my loins are full of inflammation and there is no soundness in my flesh. I am feeble and severely broken. I groan because OF THE TURMOIL OF MY HEART. Lord, all my desire is before You. My heart pants, my strength fails me. As for the light of my eyes, it also has gone from me." —*Psalm 38:6-8:*

I scared my husband so badly that he wanted to call my friends to sit with me through the day, even as Job's friends sat with him, but I said, 'please don't, they've never gone through this and they can't possibly understand how I am feeling inside.' I felt worthless. I was completely broken. I was as one who had no hope.

I didn't think I had the strength to undergo another treatment. I didn't even think I'd have the strength to get out of bed the next day. But while my husband held me and prayed I heard God speaking to me through a poem written by my friend Yolanda McElroy.

<u>Exodus</u>
Come, rise up from the dust
Virgin daughter, my beloved
Shake yourself and rise
Come and dance with me…
Your once shackled feet are now loosed…
Now rise, virgin daughter
Give glory to your God
In joy, receive liberty
Let the beauty given you
Radiate from your eyes
Raise your hands in ecstasy
As you praise the Lord Most High…

God was reminding me that I said I'd always serve him. That he'd already done enough. I could see Satan standing before the throne of God saying, 'Yeah, you've given her salvation and justification, and all these other promises, but take away her hope of having children and she'll cave. She'll stop serving you.'

Jesus had saved me. Now He was saying, **'RISE, your hope is not in this life anyway. This world is not your home. Don't run from me. Be like the prodigal son who in his distress turned back to his father-Rise, virgin daughter, my beloved…'**

But I didn't want to rise! I didn't want to stand! I wanted to wallow in my self-pity! I wanted to keep crying, 'God, I don't understand why you are being so unfair to me. I did everything right! I didn't sleep around! I cared for **Your** *children! I ministered to them and loved them.* **Why have you forsaken me?**'

I didn't want to rise. I didn't want to stand! But how could I not rise, when my mother rose. She rose while standing in the cotton field as a young girl dreaming of a better life. She rose after being taken from her home and experimented on as a child. She rose after many beatings and humiliations. She rose, though her dreams had often been crushed. She rose after a failed marriage and bitter divorce. She rose during her battle with cancer-even to the end. How could I do any less?

Still I didn't want to rise. I didn't want to stand. But my husband had prayed. He'd told me it didn't matter if we ever had children because he loved me.

God reminded me during that prayer of what I did have-gifts, talents, abilities, and a wonderful husband, who loved me unconditionally, just as my mother had. He further showed me hurting people everywhere who needed to be reminded of His goodness and grace, even in the midst of their despair.

Finally I was reminded of the greatest resurrection of all. Jesus, after being severely beaten, tormented and afflicted-for my transgressions rose! Someone did understand how I felt inside! He rose!

As the wind blew, through the leaves
I could see pieces of my soul
Bending—But I won't break...
Unless I lose my will to fight...
Excerpted from Free to Fly by Penda Horton James & Lena Arnold

So I rose, though I didn't want to rise. Though my heart was in despair and filled with anxiety for the future, I rose! I rose because I remembered that I had a high priest that had been touched with the feeling of my infirmity. God said in Psalm 138:3 and 8:

"In the day I cried out, You answered me, and made me bold with strength in my soul... The Lord will perfect that which concerns me; Your mercy, O'Lord, endures forever, Do not forsake the works of Your hands."

I remembered that God is our refuge and strength, a very present help in times of trouble, therefore we will not fear. Use your pain as an opportunity to praise God and to remember who He is, and what He promised He would do for you-for us.

What is it that torments you? What trigger causes you to become sad, depressed, or angry? I urge you to use that trigger as a catalyst to praise God, thanking Him for all that you do have. If you believe in God, then you know that Satan wants to use pain and suffering to try to interrupt our praise of God-to turn us away from Him. But when we praise God in the midst of our pain, it can no longer be used as a weapon against us. Before we know it we start to rise!

So I rose, because how else could I convince you to rise? How could I convince anyone that they are free to fly, if I had not first fallen as low as I could possibly go, and then rose? So I rose, and even in my current despair-STILL I RISE!

...You may feel cast down and forsaken. You are going through a trial different from mine, but every bit as painful to you. You hide behind fear and shame. You've endured the trite clichés and words from well meaning friends. You have borne the accusations of sin levied against you and you are tired. You feel as if you want to die, and your heart barely has the strength to go on.

But I'm here today to tell you that you can rise.

> *When (not if)* your dreams have been broken in pieces
> and your hopes appear as glass shattered
> *Remember,* it's not how you started,
> it's how you finish that matters.
> ...through the course of ... life you may falter
> the end seems nowhere in sight
> *know that...* the sun always arises,
> ...displacing the dark of the night...
> *In...life* some dreams become broken and shattered.
> ...But it's not how we start
> *It's* how we finish that matters

Rise. **Reach Inward, Seeking the Excellence of the Exalted.**

I may never have children from my own womb and if that is so I'll have to learn to live with that. You may never have all of your dreams fulfilled, and you'll have to learn to live with that. But the key is you must live. My ancestors lived with the injustice of slavery, the fear of lynching and rape.

Yet they rose! They rose because in their heart of hearts they believed there was something worth rising for. Find that thing in your life and rise!

*Though your dreams have been broken in pieces-**RISE!***
*Though your hopes appear as glass shattered-**RISE!***
*Though you falter and the end seems nowhere in sight-**RISE!***
*Though your hopes are dashed-**RISE!***
*Though your heart unleashes a torrent of tears-**RISE...***

The room was silent, and for an instant I felt alone, until I saw that everyone in the room was crying.

Women who had struggled with infertility introduced themselves to encourage me and to weep with me. Men and women in anguish over 9/11 thanked me for helping them deal with their pain. Others simply expressed their appreciation for my transparency and openness.

I needed their words and expressions of love because I had to wait two months for a cyst to resolve before attempting the next IUI. The cyst formed from my ovulation site during the previous cycle. Dr. Bidwell said this was normal, except most of the time they go away by the time your menses appears.

> *"Delight yourself also in the Lord and He shall give you the desires of your heart. Commit your way to the Lord. Trust also in Him and He shall bring it to pass."*
> **Psalm 37:4, 5**

While waiting another period came and went.

"I really feel like cussing." I told your daddy.

"I know. I feel like cussing too! Are you going to be okay?"

"I think so."

I got out of bed and showered and stayed in there so long that he yelled from the bedroom to ask if I was okay. But I was. I didn't cry or break down. This time I held no illusions. I used to keep up hope by telling myself, "Maybe I'm just spotting. It'll stop. I don't do that anymore. What it is *is* what it is and I accept it.

So I took a deep breath and said, "*God to help me praise You anyway. I know I can't even get that far without Your help. Help me fight the desire to lie down and yield myself to the pain. Give me the strength to wait on You, renew my strength and mount me up on the wings of eagles, let me run and not be weary, let me walk and not faint. Let me RISE.*"

Love Mommy

CHAPTER 6

Calling on God When Your Strength is Gone!

"Behold, children are a heritage from the Lord, the fruit of the womb is a reward."—**Psalm 127:3**

February 18, 2002

Dear Children:

"Children are a reward for what?" I asked Kim, needing someone to talk to after our third IUI attempt.

"I don't know. It gets so frustrating sometimes. I'm sick of people casually throwing away their babies like it's nothing. I just don't understand." She said.

"Hey look, I know. My cousin is on meth and my uncle is raising all of her kids, while people like you and I have to struggle. It's just not fair!"

"I mean I'm not trying to be judgmental, but… you know what I mean?"

"Well, we are both going to pray for one another that it will all work out."

"I really want this more for Craig's sake than my own. He's a great guy. I have kids, and I want him to know what it feels like to be a father."

"Let me ask you something and be straight with me." I interrupted.

"Go ahead."

"Knowing that you were the reason why you couldn't have kids, did you ever deliberately do things to push Craig to leave you so he could go be with someone who could have kids?"

"Well, no, I never did, but then Craig knew that I'd had my tubes tied and couldn't have children. But honestly I don't know what might have happened between us if we'd been in your shoes. I mean I believe Craig never would have left me but maybe I might have pushed him away."

"I think there were times when I did things to try to make Horace leave me. I guess I thought maybe he'd be better off with someone who could have his kids."

"I can see that happening. That does explain why many infertile couples don't stay together even though the non-infertile person often wants to stay married."

"Yeah," I said more to myself than to Kim.

"Look, don't worry about it, do the In-Vitro and we are going to believe God that it will work for both of us."

"You know I wasted the last two weeks being abstinent. I made the mistake of listening to my friend Kimee. 'You can't have sex because the orgasms might make you have contractions which might cause you to miscarry.' So I figured if we didn't have sex after ovulation, *assuming I was pregnant*, it would reduce that risk."

"Girl, you have got to stop playing that *Maybe If* game." Kim said.

Maybe if:
- We didn't have sex that one night…
- We'd *kept* having sex…
- I hadn't carried the laundry down the stairs…
- I hadn't mopped the floor…
- I didn't walk the dog…
- I hadn't exercised the night before my cycle…
- I hadn't drunk the prune juice…

You can always find one reason why it's your fault. And that only leads to the ANGUISH. And the anguish leads to ANGER. And the anger leads to DEPRESSION because you wonder why being a joyful mother of children doesn't apply to you.

Fortunately the depression leads you to GOD where you seek His face and He hears you and delivers you and causes you to bless Him and praise Him. And through your praise He reminds you that no matter what you are going through, no matter what enemies surround you, He is there.

> *"Because Your loving kindness is better than life, my lips shall praise You. Thus I will bless You while I live; I will lift up my hands in Your name."*
> **Psalm 63:3, 4**

And when I lift up my hands to Him I am comforted and know that no matter what, He will bring me through. As a matter of fact your daddy and I were even able to make light of the whole situation, which provided some much needed comic relief:

Tube Wars
Horace & Lena Arnold

"Okay soldiers," Said Colonel Spzoa of the Royal Guard. "We're going to need some volunteers for this mission. There will be lots of casualties, millions in fact."

"Sir, Colonel sir, may I ask a question," asked a lieutenant.

"Yes."

"What is the purpose of this mission?"

"Queen Ovary, sacred bearer of the Royal Eggs has been taken captive by the forces of Nasty Tubes and his evil henchmen. The golden eggs cannot travel down the Fallopian River. If they do not make it to their destination it is the end of humanity as we know it."

"Colonel Sir, Why can't they make it up the river?"

"No one knows. There have been no survivors from the previous missions."

"Sir..."

"No more questions."

"Sir, yes sir!"

"Do we have any volunteers? If so wave your tails. Yes I see you. You're brave soldiers. I'm not going to lie to you, it won't be easy but we will provide you with the best gear possible. To the **one or ones** who make it, there will be riches untold."

"One, only one," groaned one volunteer. "I'm outta here!"

"Sergeant Sureshot spun quickly towards him and grabbed him by the neck. "Get a hold of yourself man," he said slapping him profusely, "You're a soldier. You were born for this. Now get in there!"

"Colonel Spzoa, this is Red mission leader Captain Testy Cool, do you copy?"

"Roger that mission leader, how's it looking so far?"

"We are in the lower cervical cavity and while we have faced some hostility our soldiers are doing well. We've suffered no major casualties so far. Except for some light precipitation everything appears normal. It is dark in here so it's hard to see, Sergeant Lightswish let's get some night vision goggles out to the boys so we can get a better view of things. Colonel, I'll report back to you as we move further up the canal."

A short time later...

"Captain Testy, this is Colonel Spzoa, we haven't heard from you in a while is everything okay?"

"Sorry Colonel we faced some serious hostility as we moved further up into the Cervical Canal, can you hear me okay? We are still under heavy fire it's hard for me to hear?"

"Can you tell me what happened?"

"We put on our night vision goggles and realized that there were snipers all around us." Sound of explosions. "Oh my God, they've got land mines! Tell the boys to watch out! Colonel they are all around us, and they've got some strange chemical weaponry. When it hits us we melt!"

"Where are you now?"

"Sir we are almost at Cave Ova, where Queen Ovary is being held, but they have a fortress here. We've suffered a major blow, but I think we can make it. We still have plenty of soldiers. Captain, hold on, I've got to help out with these land mines. In the meantime send in some medics."

"No can do Captain, you're under too heavy fire, we can't risk it right now."

"You've got too COLONEL or the men will die!"

"I'll do the best I can, roger out."

Meanwhile in Queen Ovary's royal chambers…

"Your highness, we must escape through the secret Progesterone Passage now while we still have time."

"No, I cannot leave my eggs, help will come."

"But your Highness it's been twelve years. The enemy has totally taken over and will not release the eggs. He has said if we do not leave they will kill you and all your court."

"I will not leave!"

"Your highness we are running out of time!"

"They will come!"

"In 12 years no soldier has ever broken through the enemy's stronghold, and even if one did, they have barricaded the bridge to the Fallopian River and poisoned it as well. Why are you so sure that a rescuer will come?"

"The master promised he'd send a rescuer and he will come. Now leave if you want to but I must say. I will hear no more of your talk that I queen Ovary, sacred bearer if the eggs leave."

"How many more millions of soldiers will die because of your stubbornness my Queen? Nevertheless at your command I will stay."

"I know you are worried about the soldiers, but they know the risks and they willingly make the sacrifice for the sake of the One Who Will Come. They will be well rewarded for their bravery."

In the meantime the soldiers have reached the mouth of Cave Ova and are horrified by what they see.

"Colonel this is mission leader, we've reached Ova Cave and I think we are going to need reinforcements. The enemy's numbers stretches into the billions; on top of that they have barricaded the Fallopian Bridge and poisoned the river. We'll do our best, but we really need a weapon that will allow us to bypass the cave and the Fallopian River."

"Can you get to Queen Ovary and the eggs?" Asked General Spzoa.

"Well it's a funny thing, the eggs are virtually unguarded, many have been free to come and go as they please. They know the eggs are no good without their queen and her estrogen court. One of the court maidens has escaped and told us about a secret passage, but I don't know if we can make it with what we have. Is the new IVF 40 Tank available for us to use?"

"It's out on another battlefield right now and won't be available till next month; you'll have to do what you can. Get in there and tell Queen Ovary no matter what happens we will not give up! Tell your boys to get to those unguarded eggs and fertilize them!"

"Fertilize them for what Colonel, they can't get anywhere even if we get to them!"

"Look at both Fallopian Rivers, there must be a secondary access stream somewhere."

"Sir, yes sir. I'll issue the orders."

A few minutes later the Captain's earpiece is pierced by loud screams.

"Colonel, we're being ambushed. The maiden set us up."
"Red leader, this is Gold leader, do you copy?"
"I copy Gold leader, go ahead."
"I've spotted a free egg and made contact. I found a clear stream down the Fallopian River and I'm going in. I'll need some cover."
"Roger that Gold Leader."

"Colonel, this is Red leader we'll cover him."

"All right, go ahead kid."

"I'm going, I see the target, but I need cover, they're all over me– move, move, move!"

"Stay on target!"

"I'm trying, but they hit my wing!"

"Stay on target!"

"I got a shot off! Darn it missed!"

"Stay on target."

"I'm almost there!"

"Yeah!"

"Oh no!"

"What is it Gold Leader?"

"It's blocked and covered with tripwire explosives! But I'm going to try anyway."

Sound of crashing, explosives and screaming is heard.

"Mission leader this is Gold Leader, he didn't make it and all the escaped eggs have been killed! It is a terrible scene."

"Mission Leader, do you copy."

"Roger, we are under heavy fire, return to base, do you copy return to base!"

"Copy that, we are on our way!"

"Colonel this is Red Mission Leader. We have met the enemy and they are many. I don't think we are going to make it. I've given Queen Ovary your message. She assures us that she will not give up."

"What can we do," asked the Colonel?

"You've got to get the IVF Tank 40 in here, it's our only hope!"—THE END

"...Master we have toiled all the night, and have taken nothing: nevertheless at Your word I will let down the net. And when they had this done, they enclosed a great multitude of fishes; and their net brake."—Luke 5:5, 6

February 19, 2002

Dear Children:

Though I was beginning to feel like those fishermen, at Kim's encouraging words I scheduled a meeting with Dr. Bidwell the last week of January to discuss the next option in our treatment plan.

"The next logical step for you is In-Vitro fertilization. I suspect the previous IUI attempts failed because there is a problem with your tubes. The endometriosis has probably caused scarring that damaged the cilia, or thin hairs lining the tubes that move the eggs. It could also be that the tubes themselves have lost their elasticity. Now we could perform surgery to verify my suspicions, but there's no point in having you undergo another invasive procedure, when In-Vitro is the only treatment for the problem anyway."

"What do you think?" I asked Chrystal since your daddy couldn't get the time off work.

"It's your decision."

"What's your professional opinion? I mean in light of the three failed IUI's?" I asked the doctor.

"The way you responded to the medication, you seem to be a perfect candidate for it. I shared your case with our IVF Nurse Coordinator and she is excited. She loves to see numbers like yours."

"Really?"

"Yes. Some women may only produce one egg from the Clomid and you typically have at least three or more. We know you'll do well with the other medicine. If it was me, and my insurance paid for it, there would be no question for my wife and me, we'd go straight for it."

"He's right," Your dad said later that night. "We'd better take advantage of this opportunity while we can. I'm still a little apprehensive with all the ethical issues involved. I mean what if they lose our sperm or eggs?"

"What if we make more eggs than we can use? What will we do with them?" I countered.

"What if they accidentally put the wrong sperm in you, or give someone else your eggs?"

"That would be terrible, but it has happened."

"Do they use all the sperm, and if not, what happens to it?" He asked.

"Oh God, I don't know. But even before we get to that part, what if I can't handle the shots? What if it doesn't work after we've gone through all of that effort? What then? Would we be one of those couples who would have to find a surrogate?"

"Could we even bring ourselves to do that? I don't know about that, I think I'd rather adopt."

Wow! I can't believe I used to judge these couples, but now I understand the desperation that drives them. I used to judge Sarah, who urged her husband to sleep with her handmaid so he could have a child, but now I understand. Would I do that? Could I do that? I didn't want to even imagine the thought.

"You know some people are going to think we are out of God's will."

"I know. I already had that conversation with Marissa. I was telling her what we were getting ready to do and she got quiet. I asked her why she wasn't saying anything and she said, 'I'm just wondering what Jesus has to say about it. I mean I don't think In-Vitro is an acceptable option for Christians.'"

"Who asked her what she thought?"

"People feel they have a right to say something. I asked her what scriptures she was basing her word on and all she could say was '*I just don't think its right and you should seek God more.*' I told her God's Word was clear on certain matters like stealing, adultery and fornication but what's in there about this? Then I reminded her how she told me, '*you have a right to your opinion but you need to mind your own business,*' when she was talking about leaving her husband. But now that she's got an opinion for me, I'm supposed to listen. I told her that she needed to take her own advice."

"Alright, I'm glad you got with her." He applauded.

"Then she said, 'it just doesn't seem right you making a baby from your husband looking at a porno magazine. I told her my husband didn't do that, but even if he had, that was none of her business.

When I explained the process, she kept saying, 'it just doesn't seem n-a-t-u-r-a-l'."

"So I guess since aspirin isn't natural she won't take that for a headache then? Will she smoke some weed since that's natural?"

"I don't know, I didn't think of that. But I did tell her this was no different than going to the doctor to fix any other problem you might have, like heart disease, the flu, tuberculosis or any other ailment. Infertility is a physical problem and thank God that He has given doctors some answers, otherwise there'd be no hope for someone like me."

"What did she say then?"

"Well then maybe you have to be sure this is God's will."

"No she didn't! She doesn't give up. What did you say?"

"I hung up on her. I don't have time for that mess."

Sacred versus secular, faith versus science, can they really exist peacefully together? Well in the Old Testament the priests were also healers, doctors so to speak. So in the end we realize that like all the other areas of our life, we were simply going to have to trust God. We would pray and then give it to Jesus: everything, all our questions, all our fears, and all our apprehensions.

We agreed to start in March, but by Friday, Betheen the IVF Nurse Coordinator called and said that based on my last cycle we could get in on the session scheduled to begin February 4th. Within a week we were sitting in on our first education class with two other couples. There was one very nice, but nervous young couple, and one couple, with a seemingly arrogant husband. Like your daddy he also arrived late due to work, but unlike him, he came slapping his big medical book on the table and asking all these questions couched in medical vernacular. It was obvious that he was irritating the IVF Nurse because he framed many of the questions in such a way as to question her expertise. She tried her best to hide her annoyance while assuring him that she did indeed know what she was doing.

It must be pretty frustrating for him to know that he can't fix this problem by himself. In a way though I can empathize with him, engineers, like doctors want to fix things be they cars, processes, or people and I know how aggravated your dad gets when he can't fix something.

So I imagine it must be doubly annoying to be a doctor and not be able to fix your wife's infertility problem. Just the same, he could have left his self-importance at the door and swallowed his pride just like the rest of us.

Anyhow, after the customary introductions, Betheen began to explain again how the process would work.
 "In-Vitro Fertilization or IVF as we call it takes several weeks and consist of about five basic steps which includes: *ovarian follicle development, sperm collection, egg harvesting/Oocyte retrieval, In Vitro Fertilization Laboratory: and the actual embryo transfer.* Women usually grow a single egg in a month and in order to increase the chances of pregnancy occurring, we give you medication to stimulate several follicles to develop." She said. "A follicle is a bag of water that houses the egg and we monitor the egg development by performing periodic ultrasounds and checking your blood for estrogen, progesterone, and luteinizing hormone. In addition your doctor will regularly review your information in order to adequately interpret your cycle data."

The IVF team, consisting of Drs. Bidwell, Burwinkle, St.Pierre, the embryologist, and myself, evaluates these data on an ongoing basis for the appropriate timing of the administration of the human chorionic gonadotropin or HCG injection to trigger the final stages of egg maturation. The HCG injection is usually given about 35 hours before egg retrieval is scheduled."
 "How does the egg retrieval process work?" The young couple asked.

"On the day you take your HCG you will be scheduled for egg harvesting; a couple of hours before the process a sperm sample will be collected from your husband. This sample can be collected in the office or at home. If it is collected at home you will be given a special sterile condom for sperm collection. The sperm will be washed* and prepared for ovulating the eggs."

"Washed?" I asked.

"That just means the lab removes everything from the sample but the sperm."

"Oh."

"Later, you will return to the office and the eggs will be collected by transvaginal ultrasound-guided oocyte aspiration. This is a simple technique involving the introduction of a fairly small needle through the vaginal wall guided by the ultrasonic probe."

"That sounds like it might hurt." I was always concerned about pain.

"While the procedure is easy to perform there can be some pain involved. For that reason you will be given a mild intravenous sedative, as well as an analgesic."

"What happens from there?" asked the young couple.

"After that the eggs and fluid from the eggs are placed in an incubator in a special culture medium and remain in the carefully-controlled extra corporeal system for 4-6 hours before the embryologist adds the specially-processed sperm collected by your husband that morning, to allow the fertilization process to occur. In some cases we may perform ICSI to assure fertilization."

"What's ICSI?" She further questioned.

"It's a procedure where Dr. St. Pierre injects the sperm directly into the egg to ensure fertilization."

"Okay, that's interesting." Her husband remarked.

"After a period of 16-20 hours, the embryologist checks for the first signs of fertilization. If it has occurred, the embryologist should be able to observe *two pronuclei* which looks like a round ball with two eyes. These pronuclei represent the genetic material from the couple. After two to three days, if the embryos are growing normally, they are ready for the embryo transfer. The embryo transfer takes place in our office without anesthesia." She smiled at me.

"So there is no pain involved?" I asked while Betheen laughed and your daddy shook his head.

"No, other than some mild cramping, it works much like your IUI except that you'll be asked to lie still longer. The embryos are placed in a catheter and then the tiny plastic tube is introduced into the uterus through the cervix and the embryo(s) are transferred into your uterus."

"Embryos, how many are we talking about?" I questioned.

"It depends, for women younger than 35 we usually will not put in more than three, while women over 35 may have four or five placed in them. We follow guidelines set up by the Society for Reproductive Medicine. The guidelines help to reduce the risk of large scale multiple births."

"Okay." I said reassured.

As badly as I wanted kids I did not want to have five or six at one time.

"Now," she continued, "after the embryos are transferred, you will lie with your legs in the stirrups for a few minutes, then you can lie normally on your back for about an hour after the transfer.

When you get home you must be on complete bed rest for the next 24-72 hours. Even after that we ask you to restrict your physical activities until the pregnancy test."

"Does that mean she should not return to work?" The doctor's wife asked.

"Unless your job requires serious physical labor you can return to work, but no heavy lifting and no running marathons." She joked.

"Whew, this is a lot to process." The doctor's wife remarked while her husband glared at her.

"It is a lot," said Betheen. "And it can get stressful, because of that there will be a psychologist available for you to speak with whenever you need, especially if you feel overwhelmed and feel like giving up. You don't ever have to feel alone."

"So what happens after the transfer? I mean do we just sit around and wait." The young woman asked.

"After the transfer we monitor your blood levels for progesterone. Increasing levels suggest that the transfer has been successful. Two weeks from the transfer you will take a pregnancy test. If it's positive then we will continue to monitor you for 12 weeks via blood tests plus vaginal ultrasounds to detect the baby's heartbeat and determine the number of successfully implanted embryos. We usually do the ultrasound at 4 weeks."

"Wow, you can tell that soon?" Daddy and I were amazed, "I mean they must be tiny."

"Yes, they are, but the vaginal probe allows us to get right in there and take a look. It's really amazing. Every time I see it I am astounded."

"What happens if the IVF is unsuccessful?" The doctor asked in a tone that suggested it better not be.

"During a cycle we gather an enormous amount of information. In the event of an unsuccessful cycle, we schedule a meeting between you and your physician. Prior to that meeting all the information collected throughout the process is evaluated in order to plan future treatments. We may have to increase a medication, or have you take them on a different schedule. We review medication administration to ensure that it was administered correctly, with the proper dosages, and at the right times. Hopefully it all works out, but unfortunately some couples have to undergo the process more than once before a successful pregnancy occurs. Even then a successful pregnancy doesn't mean a successful delivery."

"What are your success rates?" He asked.

"Some of that depends on the age of the patient, but overall our clinics success rate is around 40%, which actually is even better than "normal" pregnancy success rates for couples without infertility issues. In general, you have a better chance of achieving a successful pregnancy through In-Vitro than if you'd tried on your own and didn't have a fertility issue. Many people are surprised when they realize that normal human reproduction is a relatively inefficient process."

"Is that right?" The young woman said incredulously.

"In a healthy couple, the probability of fertilization for any particular exposure of egg to sperm may be as high as 80%, but by the time of the first expected menstrual period after ovulation approximately one-half have miscarried. The menstrual period may not even be delayed and the couples may not even realize an early pregnancy has been lost; even then as many as one-fourth of these pregnancies end in miscarriage.

This means that the probability of a live birth, after properly timed intercourse, through one menstrual cycle, in a normally fertile couple, is thought to be no higher than 20%."

"That's interesting." I thought.

"However, in spite of these results, we must emphasize that a successful conception and childbirth cannot be guaranteed by any IVF Program. Even if the couple undergoes multiple attempts, the probability of success depends on many factors including: the woman's age (*success rates are much lower when over 38 years old*), addictions (*alcohol, smoking*) and ovarian response to the stimulating medications. Other problems can arise during IVF treatment and they include: a poor (*hormone*) response to the medication; an inability to obtain eggs due to the poor quality of the follicles; difficulties in egg retrieval, or the retrieval of poor-quality eggs which are not suitable for fertilization; or poor quality sperm the day it was collected. Be sure not to ejaculate for 2 days prior to the retrieval to ensure good quality and keep the sample as clean as possible."

"What other problems could occur?" The young man asked.

"Well, the embryos might not fertilize, and even if they do they may fail to implant when inserted. And if they do implant there is still the risk of a miscarriage or a tubal pregnancy."

"Is there any information regarding the health of In-Vitro babies?" The doctor asked.

"Other than a tendency to be born early, IVF babies have no long term health issues and are as healthy as other babies."

"Why do they tend to come early?" He asked.

"No one really knows for sure, but when they come, they are typically healthy."

"What happens if there are more embryos than can be implanted?" Daddy asked.

"Couples who have more good embryos than they can use can elect to have the extra embryos frozen for their future use. There will be consent forms to sign and an additional storage fee will be charged should it become necessary to store them. Any remaining embryos after you end IVF treatment can be stored long term, destroyed, donated to another couple, or donated for research. Nothing will happen to them without your informed consent." She paused.

"Are there anymore questions?"

"Are there any risks associated with In Vitro?" I asked.

"The injections can cause some local irritation and repeated blood testing can cause mild discomfort and bruising of the arm. The drugs may also over-stimulate the ovary and cause some pelvic discomfort due to the formation of ovarian cysts. In rare cases these drugs can cause hyper stimulation of the ovaries, in which case hospitalization and medical therapy may be needed. This rarely happens because we monitor you very carefully."

"Are there any other risks? I asked.

"The ultrasound egg retrieval procedure presents a rare possibility of infection or injury to abdominal organs or blood vessels, but again these are extremely rare." She paused. "Another risk is multiple births, but as I said before, limiting the number of embryos implanted minimizes this possibility, at the most you may have twins. Are there any more questions?" When no one answered she said, "Okay, let's learn to use your medication."

Betheen was very organized and handed each couple a custom notebook of information that included individualized calendars of our injection schedules, appointments, and tentative retrieval and transfer dates; all that was followed by a video on how to mix and administer the medications.

Then she gave us the opportunity to practice mixing the medicine as well as to ask more questions.

At any rate, two days after the education session I received my medicine via Fed Ex; a box full of hormone medicine, needles, instructions, alcohol wipes, etc. I was like, "Oh my goodness! I can't believe I'm really doing this!"

This is the beginning of the third week of the process and I'm up to two shots per day. It really didn't start getting sore until I had to switch to the bigger needle for the Gonal F and Repronex. I was totally unprepared for just how hard this would be. The prayer and exercise has helped reduce the stress, but nothing has alleviated the soreness in my stomach from the daily injections.

Betheen told us that if we get too sore in our stomach to switch to our thighs. Oh boy, that hurts worse than the stomach! I'm not looking forward to the intramuscular injections of progesterone at all!

I remember telling Bonita, that God would never put me through this because He knows I couldn't deal with shooting myself in the stomach. Yet here I am.

"Lord You made me, now give me the strength to endure what I never thought possible."

Love Mommy

"All Dogs Go To Heaven"
Disney Movie

February 27, 2002

Dear Children:

Ivan died this week and I've been crying everyday since.

In between all that I had to make numerous visits to the doctor for ultrasounds and blood draws. The following Monday I went to the clinic for my last ultrasound before the retrieval. Doctor Bidwell was excited, "It appears that the medicine really took effect. It looks like we'll get eight good ones, maybe even 12." He said excitedly.

I was told to take my HCG shot later that night around 11 P.M. Based on my previous ultrasound they moved the retrieval and transfer back one day, which worked out well because your daddy would only have to take one day off work. The transfer will take place on March 2nd and I'm so excited!

That exhilaration was almost destroyed this morning after looking at the sample we'd gathered. "It's all smushed, it can't be any good." I cried!

After we dropped off it off at the lab, Betheen led me back to the exam room to change and start my I.V. "I'm so excited for you guys! This is going to be great!"
    "Are you sure? I don't know if our sperm sample was good enough."
    "It was fine."

Your dad helped me change into my gown, and then Dr. Bidwell came in to talk to us. A few minutes later they took me to another room by the lab, got me situated on the table/chair-whatever they call that thing, with my legs all up in the air, then started the I.V.

Within five minutes I began drifting off, though I knew what was going on around me. I could hear talking as they collected each egg. After a few minutes they let your daddy in.

Dr. Bidwell returned to tell us the total number of eggs they collected.
"Most of them were immature, four are perfect."
"Oh, no," I groaned inwardly, not wanting to go through this again.
"We're going to allow the immature ones to remain in the culture an extra day. We'll keep you informed of how they are progressing, and Dr. St. Pierre will take pictures of the embryos for you once they are fertilized. You will get to see your babies in a way most people never do–at conception!" I was still too drowsy to fathom the magnitude of it all.

God told Adam and Eve to, "Be fruitful and multiply, replenish the earth and subdue it." That story got me to thinking about Jesus. To me, IVF proves Jesus' conception and birth. Think about it! If man, created in the *image* of God can take a man's sperm, extract a woman's egg, fertilize them in a dish, and re-implant them into a woman, then why is it so hard to believe that God the *Creator* can implant His essence/His Spirit/His Self, into a woman's egg and create a baby?

This process has also made me think about Gideon, God repeatedly reduced the number of warriors called to battle till their number was so small that they should have been destroyed by their foes, but they won the battle with only a few hundred men. This process is His great testimony for our lives!

> *"...Contentment is one of the flowers of heaven, and if we would have it, it must be cultivated...It cost him (Paul) some pains to attend to the mystery of that great truth..."*—**Charles H. Spurgeon**

God is my contentment and my peace. He will take what seems to be weak to us and work a miracle.

Love Mommy

"My flesh and my heart fail; But God is the strength of my heart and my portion is forever."—***Psalm 73:26***

March 5, 2002

Dear Children:

"Your brother and sister-in-law aren't getting any younger. It's about time they got started." That's what he said to me. He shall remain nameless for reasons of familial, i.e. political correctness.
"It's not that easy for everyone to have children you know." I said.
"I mean I don't know what they are waiting on. Man they've been married longer than you guys haven't they?"
"Yeah, so get a clue," I thought.
"They're going to be all old when their kids get here…"
"Age ain't nothin' but a number on your driver's license," I said. "It's really not that easy for everyone, you know what I mean? C'mon, you're a smart guy; you must know what I'm trying to say."

Thank God smart people also say good things too.
"Lena I envy you." Janet said.
"What? Why in the world would you envy me?"
"People typically take for granted being able to have a baby through the *normal* process may never experience God the way you and Horace have. A struggle like that can only bring you closer to God."
"Hmm, I've never thought about it that way before. We have learned to trust Him in a way I'd never thought possible and learned so much about real faith and real trust." I said.

I mean I'm laying flat on my back writing in a journal to children who don't exist. Oh, that reminds me, I guess I should tell you why I'm on my back.

Since I last wrote, 4 of the 15 eggs they collected at the retrieval fertilized properly into embryos, but one of the four didn't make it. I felt like having a funeral, but how do you do that?

Of the 11 that remained, seven of them matured and were fertilized through rescue ICSI (Intracytoplasmic sperm injection.) All that means is that they assisted fertilization by shooting the sperm directly into each egg. Of those, three fertilized properly for a total of six, but by Saturday one of them failed to split, leaving only five fertilized embryos to implant.

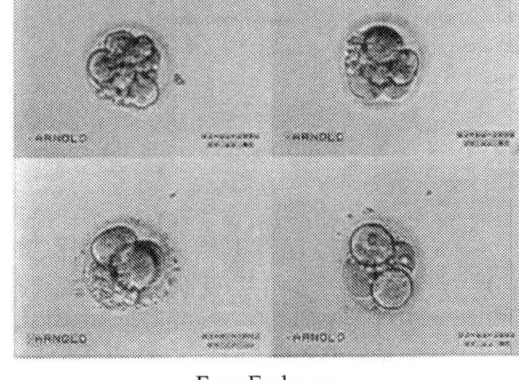

Four Embryos

I'd hoped to have enough to freeze, so I wouldn't have to go through the entire process over again, but Betheen encouraged me.

"Many people don't have this many. All things considered, you did very well. You had a great response to the medicine."

Prior to the procedure they gave us the final count and asked us if we wanted them to implant all five. Normally, for a woman of my age they would implant no more than four, but one of the embryos was splitting slowly and they felt it had a better chance of survival in my womb, rather than undergoing freezing and storage.

You should have seen the look in your daddy's eyes at the thought of all five actually surviving! All he could think about was how he was going to feed five babies?"

"What should we do?" I said looking at Betheen.

"Go for it." She nodded. "With five implanted you have a greater chance of knowing at least one will take."

I always wanted at least four kids, but now I could be having five at once! I looked at daddy, he shook his head yes, and I said, "Let's do it."

Your dad was a great coach, helping to keep me calm because my bladder felt like it was about to burst. I couldn't go to the bathroom because a full bladder gave them superior view of the uterus.

The procedure was much like the IUI, except that Dr. St. Pierre verified that no embryos were left in the transfer catheter. The room was set-up so that air could only flow one way to maintain sterility. It was cool how you could watch the whole process on a monitor. They even gave us a picture of the actual implant. I had to take their word for it, because to me it just looked like a comet in the sky.

"Now, whatever you do, resist the temptation to take a pregnancy test before we administer one. It won't give you a false negative, but it could give you a false positive..." She didn't have to finish. I knew what she meant. A false positive might have me all geeked up, only to be let down. The blood test would be far more conclusive than the urine test.

"I'll wait." I promised.

Before I knew it they were done. And just like after the IUI I had to lay flat for a while, except this time I also had to go home and stay flat in the bed for a couple of days. That's what I'm doing now, laying low and trying my best not to think more about this than I should.

It didn't seem like a blessing during all the years of waiting, but now I realize that Janet was right. Through this process I have peeked into the heart of God. No matter what happens to these little embryos I believe that I have five children, even if I only see them on the other side.

All we can do now is wait and I am discovering that this wait is as difficult as the previous one.

"...God considers how we handle the wait as important as what we are waiting for..." (Sandra Glahn & William Cutrer M.D.)

    "Waiting is the hardest," said a patient interviewed by Dr. Cutrer for the book *"When Empty Arms Become A Heavy Burden: Encouragement for couples Facing Infertility,"* "...I just want to

> get it over with so that I can know what I am dealing with and try to live normally again for a few brief weeks... you put your life on hold and have to act as though you are already pregnant...you can't do anything strenuous so that your precious embryos may implant firmly...for two weeks you have to pretend you're pregnant, being careful not to get carried away with the fantasy of it all."

I know exactly what she's talking about. But during those two weeks it feels good to pretend being special, all the while knowing it could end at any moment.

> *"Weeping may endure for a night, but joy comes in the morning."*
> **Psalm 30:5**

Yet I refuse to accept that God brought us through all this to leave us. We asked Him to give us enough embryos to have a successful implant, but not so many that we'd have to decide what to do with them. God honored that request, so why wouldn't He honor the rest? I have to believe that the end will be sunshine and rejoicing. The Lord will perfect that which concerns me!

God understands me, meaning He <u>stands under me</u>, carrying me when I can no longer go on my own. He lifts me up and affirms me, all the while upholding my humanity.

William Quale said, *"March is the trumpet month, the jubilant month. March winds do not blow trumpets for fun. That is their business, which they stick to with astonishing fidelity...stormy winds come not without blessing. There is music in the blast if we listen closely. Watch the winds transform into a boisterous lover of flowers and the spring leaf."*

Love Mommy

CHAPTER 7

Praising God In the Sunshine!

"I WAITED patiently for the Lord; He inclined unto me, and heard my cry. He brought me up also out of a horrible pit, out of the miry clay, and set my feet upon a rock...he has put a new song in my mouth, even praise unto our God: Many shall see it and fear, and shall trust in the Lord."—**Psalm 40:1-3**

Friday, March 15, 2002

Dear Children:

"Do you really think I have brought you this far to leave you?"

"No," I heard my voice say, "but it would be nice to know for sure."

As I pulled into the hospital parking lot I heard a radio program about a group of college students who'd gone rafting down a river after they had been warned not to go down.

Their raft capsized and one of them got trapped on an island in the middle of the river, so he started praying. Another got trapped in a whirlpool. While another escaped and managed to get help for the others. But by the time help arrived the one in the whirlpool had been trapped underwater for 45 minutes. Miraculously he survived– *with no brain damage*!

Each thanked God for His mercy in spite of the fact that they'd ignored the warnings. Lord, if You can do that for them, You can do it for me, I said to myself, gaining the courage I needed to take the pregnancy test.

Afterwards I went back to work, but left early, knowing I would not be able to hang in there all day with my nerves so up in the air. When I arrived home there was a message on the answering machine from Betheen. I got concerned, because "Betheen is normally off on Friday's. Is the news so bad that everyone else is afraid to tell me? Or is it *so good* that she wants to tell me herself?
    "Oh just call and get it over with." I said to myself.

She wasn't in, but they promised to have her get in touch with me as soon as possible. "Oh, no," I thought, trying my best not to read too much into it. I was in the bedroom sitting in the chair trying to stay relaxed when the phone rang. I snatched it up quickly.

"Hello," trying my best to sound nonchalant.

"Lena," It was Betheen. "I have good news for you..." I started screaming before she could finish. There was so much joy that I promise you I could feel her smile over the phone.

"YOU'RE PREGNANT!"

"Raise a song and strike the timbrel, the pleasant harp with the lute."
Psalm 81:2

After two weeks of being on edge, 12 years of being married, and 16 years of being together you are finally on the way!

"Your HCG level was 381." She said excitedly. "That's very good. You'll have to have a second test on Monday, but don't worry. You are pregnant!"

"Oh, thank you Jesus!" I cried tears of joy. Thank you! Thank you guys so much."

"Hey, you guys did all the work." She said happily.

"Oh no, no, no, this was a joint effort. You guys are AWESOME!!!!

I am so happy! Thank you so much for calling me yourself, for a minute I was scared thinking maybe everyone else was afraid to tell me the news because it was bad."

"Are you kidding, it was all they could do not to say anything when you called. I made them promise not to because I wanted to tell you myself."

"You are so sweet!" I'd liked her from the beginning and I liked her even more now.

"Well thank you." I could feel her smile over the phone, "Make sure you call the office on Monday to schedule your next appointment. We won't know for sure how many implanted until your ultrasound at four weeks."

"Wow, four weeks and you can tell that much that soon?"

"Yes, performing a vaginal ultrasound allows us to see things earlier than the conventional ultrasound. You'll stay with us for the next 12 weeks before we release you back to your OB/GYN. Okay, so don't forget."

"Oh I won't. Thank you Betheen, and please thank Drs. Bidwell, Burwinkle, and St. Pierre for me. I really appreciate you guys."

"I'll tell them; in the meantime you guys have a great weekend and again congratulations!"

> God heard our cry and answered every desire of our heart
> He comforted us when we felt worthless and cast down
> He caused us to laugh, to run, to RISE
> He captured our tears, saved them, and kept them near.
> In the day of His choosing He received them
> And spread blessings to His people

Your dad was ecstatic! We made plans to celebrate later that evening. Janet was hyped!

"I knew it when you told me you couldn't sleep and that you were constantly running to the bathroom." Dana said.

You are due around Thanksgiving and when I think of all the Thanksgiving's I've spent depressed this is poetic justice.

Love Mommy

"For I have known him, in order that he may command his children and his household after him, that they keep the way of the LORD, to do righteousness and justice, that the Lord may bring to Abraham what He has spoken to him."—Genesis 18:19

April 24, 2002

Dear Children:

Its official, in this photo you are one-month gestation. Your little heart is beating, see!

I had my first ultrasound on March the 27th to determine how many babies we are actually going to have.

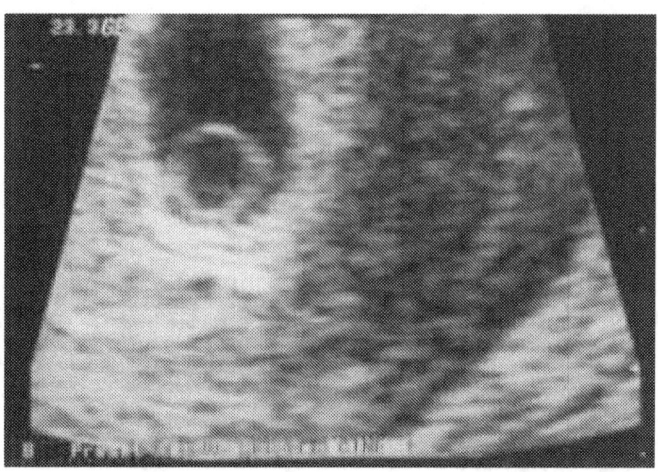

So far there are two. One is developing a lot slower so they were unable to see much. Dr. Bidwell doesn't think the smaller one will survive, but we are praying that by the time we go back in two weeks things will look better.

I couldn't actually see your heart because it was so tiny, but I saw the repeated *blip, blip, blip* from a tiny spot on the edge of the yolk sac. It was captivating!

We're definitely going to do this again, although, according to Dr. Bidwell I could get pregnant on my own because pregnancy will temporarily stop the endometriosis, allowing my body time to heal from the previous damage.

Who would've thought that all those years ago? I never thought I'd be able to handle it.

"Five babies, how are you going to take care of five babies?" My former co-worker remarked.

Why is she trying to rain on my parade?

"Why ya'll wanna have kids now, your life is about to be over." Daddy's brother said.

Our life is being renewed!

"Dude, you're an old man now, I mean 36 is kinda old to be having a baby." My brother said.

"How old would you be if you didn't know how old you were?" —Satchel Paige said!

"Our kids are almost grown and you're just now having babies, boy I am glad I'm not you." Another friend said.

I'm glad I'm me!

On April 3rd, morning sickness kicked in and contrary to the name it can last all day. I read somewhere that the nausea could be caused by the increase in progesterone and its effects on the stomach. I'm probably getting a double dose because I'm still taking the shots.

"Why are you still taking the progesterone shots?" Tina asked.

"They have me taking it as an insurance policy. Apparently it's naturally produced in the ovaries during pregnancy. It thickens the lining and keeps it from shedding."

"Well if your body already produces it why do you need more?"

"If a woman's body doesn't produce enough it could cause a miscarriage, so the doctors typically have fertility patients take it throughout the 12th week of pregnancy. Honey I don't think I can last that long. My hips are sore and swollen.

They gave me a vaginal cream to use, but when they warned me not to let it get impacted I decided to go back to the shots."

"Impacted, like all stuck together inside you?"

"Yeah, I guess, that sounds gross doesn't it?"

"Girl you ain't lying."

"My hips are starting to hurt more and Horace is running out of places to shoot me where I have not already been stuck dozens of times."

"Oh, that does not sound like fun."

"It isn't. Besides being sore from the shots I was at home sick all day on my birthday, and the vomiting followed. I can't eat anything sweet!"

"*YOU* can't eat sweets? Girl you must be sick!"

"I know and can you believe that I've had no desire for my two favorite things, chocolate and ice cream."

"Oh no, I can't believe that!"

"I'm telling you I can't eat it. Yesterday I was feeling well enough to go to the drive-in with Mark & Dana. I even ate a snickers bar. I can't wait for it to be over so we can start hitting the garage sales."

"Girl, I already picked up something. I couldn't wait." She said. "I'm going to bring it over today."

"Can you believe I was afraid that laughing; coughing and sneezing would harm the baby?" I said.

"That's not really silly. I would probably be a little scared too those things would cause a miscarriage."

I saw you again on April 10th. See, there you are. You're bigger and though you were only about 2-3 centimeters the doctor could tell what was your head.

This miracle of modern technology takes my breath away. At four weeks we could see you and watch your heartbeat via the vaginal ultrasound, and progress your growth only two weeks later.

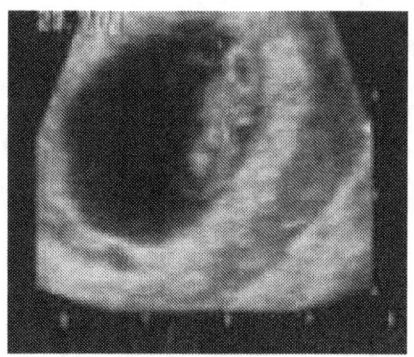

Eight weeks gestation

I mean you are tiny, but you are definitely there and you are remarkable!

Love Mommy

I try 2 picture my life
W/O U Lord
I get a feeling inside
Like I'm at war...
I try 2cry when I fall
U pick me up Lord...
When my life spins 2a stall
U keep me movin' Lord...
U are my all in all
U are my Lord...

May 26, 2002

Dear Children:

"Horace!" I screamed to your daddy during my middle of the night bathroom run. He jumped up out of bed thinking someone was trying to break into the house.

"What's wrong?"

"I'm bleeding!" I cried staring at the scary looking blood clot.

"Oh no," he groaned, trying to be strong for my sake.

"What should I do?" I asked nervously.

"I don't know, but I know how to pray." We returned to bed and I opened up, *What To Expect When You're Expecting* to see what I should do. I wasn't cramping, nevertheless the book suggested I call the doctor.

"Hi Lena, I got your message. What's going on?" Dr. Bidwell asked.

"I'm sorry to bother you, but I was bleeding and I didn't know what to do."

"It's no problem at all. Are you cramping?"

"No, I don't think so."

"What color is the blood?"

"It's bright red. And there was some clotting. One was pretty big."

"Does it seem to have slowed or stopped?"

"I don't think it's any worse than before I called. But I don't know for sure." I said trying my best to hide my fear. "Well now that you mention it, it does seem to have stopped." That helped calm me down.

"That's good. I want you to take two ibuprofens. That will help to relax the uterus and stop any contractions that may be occurring. I also want you to drink plenty of liquids and try to relax.

Come into the office the first thing in the morning. I'll do an ultrasound to check and make sure everything is alright." I tried to go back to sleep, but neither of us really slept much after that.

I arrived at the office as soon as they opened. Doctor Bidwell asked me how I was holding up. I told him okay, but the truth is I was on the brink of breaking down right then and there. I was heartsick. I wanted to believe you were okay, but until I could see you moving again, I was scared. As soon as he put the probe in we saw you move and we were both reassured.

"See right there?" He said, pointing to the upper left hand side of the screen. "It's what I suspected. A small area of the placenta has dislodged from the uterus."

"That sounds kinda bad."

"It can be, but the good news is that this sort of thing usually repairs itself as the uterus grows. The bad news is that you'll have to be on restricted activity and bed rest for the next five days or more. We'll check you again on the 7th to see how it's going." Suddenly the nausea was a small inconvenience.

For You will light my candle: the Lord my God will enlighten my darkness.
For by You I have run through a troop;
and by my God I have leaped over a wall."
Psalm 18:28, 29

"Hey girl, what's going on? I meant to call you before I went out of town, but I wasn't able." Janet asked. "Is everything okay?"

"Yes. Why do you ask?"

"Well, never mind, as long as you're okay."

"I did have something scary happen Thursday morning. I tried to call you, but I forgot you were going out of town."

"Oh boy!"

"I'm fine though."

"Okay, it's just that early Thursday morning I had this terrifying dream that you lost the baby and I had to be the one to tell you"

"You what?"

"It seemed so real and it scared me so bad that it woke me up in a cold sweat. "God, please don't let this happen. Not after all this." I prayed.

"Are you serious?" I asked.

"Yeah, that's why I asked you if everything was okay. I was so afraid I was going to get back in town and hear some bad news."

"WOW! You almost did!" I started crying.

"What happened?" She asked.

"You won't believe this, but early Friday morning about 3 A.M. I woke up bleeding."

"Oh, no, are you for real?"

"Yeah girl, I 'bout scared Horace to death. A part of my placenta had broken off. I'll be on bed rest at least until Tuesday, maybe longer."

"I'm so glad I didn't call you before I left then because I really would have scared you. Man, thank God for that dream because I'm serious I was really praying."

God's word says, when the enemy comes in like a flood, the Spirit of the Lord will lift up a standard against him." When we can't see God, He still sees us.

> *When in darkness we walk,*
> *Nor feel the heavenly flame,*
> *Then is the time to trust our God*
> *And rest upon His name.*
> *A.M. Toplady*

Love Mommy

> You are-A gift from God
> You are-A special child
> You are-The one God's created to be
> Something more than what you are...

June 1, 2002

Dear Children:

I'm almost 12 weeks along this and this is my last visit to the fertility clinic. My emotions are mixed. Leaving means I am well enough to go back to my regular OB-GYN, but it also means I am leaving my weekly support.

We were the last appointment of the day. Dr. Bidwell asked, "So how are you doing today? I hope better than the last time."

"Pretty good, much better than before."

"Feeling okay?"

"Okay I guess, except for the nausea."

"Yeah, that's the unfortunate side effect of pregnancy." He laughed. "Is it normal, or does it seem excessive?"

"I guess it's pretty normal."

"By the way, is there a formal term for what happened to me a few days ago?" I was curious, so I asked.

"Well," he slowed, "you actually had a threatened miscarriage."

"Do you think it could happen again?" I gasped.

"It could, but I seriously doubt it. Your placenta is getting pretty thick and it looks like it is much better than that day. Let's check everything out and see how the baby is doing and I'll be able

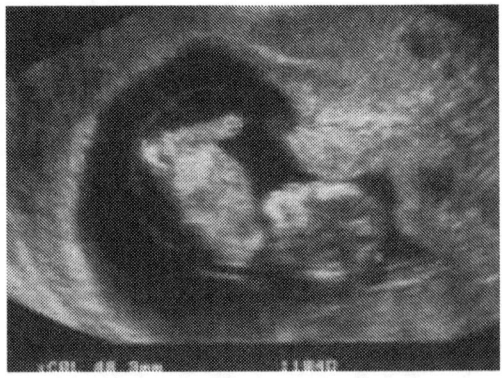

11 Weeks Five Days

to reassure you even more."

He performed the ultrasound and we were all thrilled. You had gained some weight and we could see you better.

"The baby's got a strong heartbeat. That's good."

"I notice it seems to be slower with each progressive ultrasound."

"That's normal. Typically as the baby grows the heart rate slows down. By the time the baby is born the heart will beat at about 120 beats per minute."

"Oh," we said.

"Dr. Watson is really excited about your pregnancy."

"Really?"

"Oh yes, he can't wait to see you. He was just grinning from ear to ear when I saw him."

"He's a great guy, a great doctor. I thank God he sent me to you guys."

"Yes, he is. Well, do you guys have any questions for me?"

"Yes, I do," said your dad. "Would you tell her that having sex, sneezing, doing laundry, or walking up and down the stairs is not going to harm this baby?"

"Oh yeah, you can do all those things."

"Work with me Doc." I said. He laughed.

"Obviously you have to use judgment and discretion with regard to activities, but I can safely say having sex will not harm the baby."

He continued, "Things are looking so well in fact, that I'm going to go ahead and release you back to Dr. Watson. Initially I thought I might have to keep you past the 12 weeks, but you're doing great. Have you scheduled an appointment with him yet?"

"Yes."

"Good, he's going to be really happy to see you. If you don't have any more questions, you are officially released."

It was a strange feeling being released. I didn't like it at all. After so much intimacy it didn't feel right just walking away. I mean I knew it had to happen sooner or later, but I would not only miss the staff, who'd labored so hard on our behalf, but the weekly ultrasounds that verified that the pregnancy was progressing normally. And I would miss watching you grow over the remaining six months.

Now, I have to process this feeling of being pregnant on my own. I mean its great being pregnant, but it still feels kind of weird. Like I don't know where I belong. I've been infertile for so long, that as great as these clothes feel, it doesn't seem as if they are mine.

People congratulate me for being pregnant and I can hardly thank them because I think to overly express my happiness is to betray my comrades fighting against infertility. People just assume it came easy and I want to tell them what we went through, but they didn't ask for all that information.

"Boy, they really seem like they have it *going on over there*." Our new neighbor said to Theresa. His wife's pregnant, she stays at home, and they have that shiny new vehicle. It must be nice."

"You don't have a clue as to what they have been through." She responded irritated.

"You can't just look over somebody's fence and decide without knowing them that their world is so much better than yours. They struggled over the years with all types of issues, so they deserve everything good that is happening to them now!"

You tell them Theresa!

The following week your Grandma drove to Yellow Springs with me to see Dr. Watson. Just as Dr. Bidwell had said, Dr. Watson was excited. "I told you we'd get you pregnant." He said smiling as he entered the room.

"You did, didn't you?" I smiled back.

"Where's the man at?" He took my hand and patted.

"He's at work. He doesn't' have much vacation time left so he figured he'd better save it until we get closer to when I am due."

"That's a good idea. So how are you feeling? Are you excited?"

"We are ecstatic! It's like a dream you know, after all this time it still hardly seems real!"

"It's real alright. I was so excited when Dr. Bidwell told me."

"That's what he said. I'm telling you, you guys are awesome."

"Well, we try, but I told you, didn't I? I told you my guys would get you pregnant!" He beamed excitedly.

"And words can never adequately express my appreciation to you all either."

"Awww, you stop it!" He smiled some more. "Well let's check things out, I'll be back after you get changed." When he left the nurse came in excitedly. She took my vitals, a urine sample, and drew some blood. She dug into my arms trying to find a good vein before finally calling in another who thankfully got it on the first try.

The check up was more than a notion. I was poked, prodded, and pressed in/on every body part I have. I was still walking funny a week later! The only part of the exam I enjoyed was listening to your heartbeat.

"Are you taking prenatal vitamins?"

"I was, but I ran out."

"I'm going to write you a prescription for a prenatal vitamin, make sure you take them. Otherwise you're doing great. Congratulations, I am so happy for you, and again, I hope you have a girl."

"Why do you want me to have a girl?"

"Girls are fun." He laughed,

"Tell Horace I'm sorry I missed him, but I hope to see him next time."

"I will. You have a great day and thanks again Dr. Watson."

"My pleasure."

In spite of the morning sickness I'm really starting to enjoy being pregnant. People treat you differently. Men actually make a point of opening doors for you, instead of acting like they don't see you! It's great!

The only downside to it all is that my mom is not here to enjoy it with me. I really miss her. I can't tell her how much I treasure her wisdom.

Love Mommy

"..., giving thanks always for all things to God the Father in the name of our Lord Jesus Christ..."—**Ephesians 5:19, 20**

July 4, 2002

Dear Children:

"So, how are you feeling?" Tracee asked, as we watched the men prepare for the fireworks show at your grandma's.

"I'm pretty good right now. I have been having some serious morning sickness, but usually by this time of the day I feel better. I told my aunts I wasn't getting big fast enough. Then the other day I took a really good look at myself in the mirror and realized I AM HUGE! And I am not finished growing yet! I think I look like a fat cow, but Horace loves it."

"Girl you are funny," she laughed.

"My butt's bigger, my breasts are bigger, and my belly — we won't even go there!" Tracee cracked up. "I must have been in serious denial."

"Have you felt the baby moving yet?"

"Not yet, but according to the books I should be feeling something soon. We have an ultrasound coming up and we'll find out then what we are having."

"You want to know?"

"Yeah, after waiting all this time I want to know."

"I am just so excited for you guys!"

"I know it's been such a long time coming. I can't wait for you guys."

"Me either." She said. I'm glad we can talk about it though.

"It's so needed, especially in the church. It's something nobody really wants to deal with, you know? Too many of us are suffering alone, not knowing that there are others who are just like us. I mean, look at our family for example. Speaking of that where are you guys in all this?"

"Well, we never seem to be on the same page, either he's totally ready and I'm not, or I'm totally ready and he's not, most of the time he won't even talk about it. He just believes it will happen when it happens."

"You guys have been married longer than us; it's not likely that it's just going to happen. It's time for the two of you to get serious about looking into the root cause of your infertility. I hate that we waited so long."

"I know I regret that we did not seek answers sooner, especially since my doctor fears early menopause might be setting in."

"Dr. Watson was worried about that with me as well. You guys should go see him." I said.

"Get me the number." She said. "I know I need to call somebody."

"Even if you don't call him, call somebody."

"We have to do something before I hurt someone because if one more person says something stupid to me, girl I don't know what I am going to do." I smiled, totally understanding.

"I'm so tired of people telling me how old we will be by the time our kids get out of high school. Or saying to us *'I'm glad we got our kids out of the way when we were young, now I can have some fun.'*"

"Time is only relative to how much of it you have left. Shoot, my grandma had her last baby at 45, and she lived to be 89." I said.

"You are absolutely right. I'm still young. And we intend to have fun when our kids come." I nodded in agreement.

"That's right. Years ago I prayed that if God was going to give us children later in life that He would make Horace like Joshua and Caleb. Eighty years old and kicking butt!"

"I hear you!"

"Lord mold us, shape us, and prepare us to be parents. Our job is to wait on You and Yours is to answer the prayer. I trust that as we commit our ways to You, You will bring it to pass."

Love Mommy

> *"...whatsoever is lovely, whatever is admirable...*
> *if anything is excellent or praiseworthy, think about such things..."*
> **Philippians 4:8**

July 5, 2002

Dear Children:

"According to your pre-test you are at risk for delivering a down syndrome child," she said. We had to see the other doctor in the practice today. "Have you decided about the amniocentesis?"

"They told me it would come back abnormal because of my age. Was it abnormal in some other way?" I asked.

"It doesn't look like it, but you really might want to consider having it done."

"What are the risks of having the procedure?"

"The risks are minimal, but there is a 5% chance of miscarriage."

"If she has the amniocentesis and it comes back positive, what can you do about it?" Chrystal asked.

"We'll there's really nothing that can be done. Some parents just like to know in advance."

"Knowing the risks, and knowing that there's nothing that can be done if the test comes back positive, why would I want to have it done?"

"Well, some parents like to have time to come to grips with it and prepare. Others may want to make a decision about continuing the pregnancy."

I was now more than five months pregnant, had seen my baby from the beginning of life, heard its heartbeat, and felt it moving.

I knew she meant well, but as a board member of a local non-profit benefiting special needs children and I'd come to appreciate the unique creations of God they were. Not one parent among this group would trade their special children for all the money in the world.

I know people have them everyday, and most of the time they turn out okay, but my cousin's turned out badly. She almost lost her child when her uterus kept leaking weeks after her procedure. With all that I endured to have this baby, there was no way I was allowing someone to stick a long needle in my belly and drain some of the precious fluid that was sustaining it's life, even if there was only a 5% chance of miscarriage. It was too great a risk! No, as the scripture says I will focus on what is just, pure, lovely, and of good report.

"No, I'm not going to have it." I finally said, "You can't fix the problem, and knowing this far in advance really wouldn't help me anymore than knowing later. The risk, though small, is still too great for me. I'm not minimizing the procedure, nor will I judge any woman who elects to have it. It just isn't for me."

"Okay," She smiled, "I just wanted you to have all the information. If you are okay with your decision I'll go ahead and schedule your ultrasound."

"God, there are many women who will elect to have this procedure, because they want to be able to prepare in advance for their special child; regardless of the reasons for their decision I pray that you will bless them, be with them, and keep their babies safe."

Love Mommy

*"Therefore take no thought for the morrow:
for the morrow shall take thought for the things of itself..."*
Matthew 6:34

August 29, 2002

Dear Baby Girl:

After a morning of multi-tasking I met up with Tina at the manicurist parlor where Dawn works. Her shop is at Ned's (and I'm not kidding) Car Wash/Beauty Shop/Manicure Parlor.

It's like comedy central up in there. In this one building you can have your hair cut and styled, get your nails manicured and have your feet pedicured; all while waiting for your car to be washed and detailed. Plus I heard he's going to re-open the restaurant next door and sell dinners.

So you will be able to "git yo *hur'* did, yo' *nails* did, yo' *cur' warshed*, and eat ribs all at the same time! It's a trip, like your sitting in the movie *Barbershop,* only there's a car getting washed on the other side of the window!

While I was there some guys kept ogling me. You wouldn't believe how many times I've been hit on since I've been pregnant; more in the last two months than in my whole 12 years of marriage. It's flattering, but at the same time kind of scary because I've heard there are men who are ONLY into pregnant women. That's a little bit 'o strange.

Anyway, I digress again. Dawn was finishing up Chrystal when Tina and I arrived. "You look good considering you're having a girl." She said.
  "Thanks, I think."
  "No, I mean it. Girls take your beauty and boys give you beauty."
  "I don't know about that, but this girl sure does make me sick."

"Oh really now!" Tina said sarcastically.

"You know what I mean."

"All things considered," Dawn continued, "pregnancy is really working for you."

"Thanks, other people have told me that too, but I'd hate to see what I'd look like if it wasn't working for me."

"When I was pregnant, I went from a 36 D to a 42 KKK. Do you realize how big that is?"

"It's incredulous! Three K's in the same sentence can't be good for anybody."

"It's FREAKISH!" She exclaimed, not connecting with my poor excuse for a pun.

"Right after my son was born my milk came in; I hope that does not happen to you. I had to have a special bra made before they would let me leave the hospital. Then on top of that, my milk ducts got clogged! I was in so much pain."

"See that's why I couldn't breast feed," Tina said. "It hurt too much."

"You only tried it once. You never gave yourself time." I reminded her.

"No, that was too much, I wasn't having it."

"I eventually developed benign tumors and had my breast reduced at the same time they removed my tumors." Dawn was uninterrupted,

"That does not sound like fun."

"It wasn't." She changed gears, "So are you going to breastfeed?"

"I was until I heard your story," I laughed.

"It's good if you can, it's best for the baby."

"Are you going natural?"

"Yeah right," Chrystal chimed.

"What do you mean natural? If you mean natural as in the baby is coming through my vagina, then yes. But if you mean natural as in without the use of drugs, then no way."

"I had Chris natural and it wasn't so bad." Chrystal said, "It was like having menstrual cramps, but ten times worse. I mean it hurt, but when it was over I felt good. I got up, took a shower, and didn't have much pain."

"I went natural too." Tina said.

"I know, and I still can't believe that." I replied.

"I ain't gonna lie though, I probably would have taken the drugs, but by the time I wanted them I was dilated too far and I couldn't have them."

"You did well though. You were much tougher than I ever thought. That's why I was surprised after going through all that you couldn't handle the pain of breast feeding."

"I know."

"Horace wants me to go natural if I can."

"Girl ain't nothing natural about being in all that pain." Dawn said.

"Horace ought to know better than that." Chrystal said.

"I don't know I told him I'd try."

"You know good and well you are going to take those drugs." She said.

"You know good and well I am." I laughed. "Especially if its ten times worse then menstrual cramps, you know I can barely deal with them."

"You can do it. With God all things are possible." Chrystal said.

"Everything but that!" We laughed and had a good time talking till around seven and I could not take anymore. "I'M HUNGRY!"

"Didn't you just eat an hour ago?" Dawn laughed, "It's a good thing I'm finished."

"That was just a snack and I'm glad you're done because I don't think I can take it anymore."

We all headed our separate ways. I ordered a pizza on the way home and I later wished I hadn't because it turned out to be awful. I got home around 8:15 and noticed the car wasn't in the driveway. I tried not to be nervous since I had had been trying to call your daddy since 5:30. I came in the house and checked the voice mail and when there was no message I started to get worried because your daddy always calls.

By 9:20 I decided that I would pretend to have called the police and reported him as missing. Soon as I had the thought he came walking through the door. I gave him the look.

"What?"

"If you ever leave this house without leaving me a note or calling you are gonna get it."

"You'll have to catch me first pregnant lady." He laughed while running away from me.

"That's not fair. I'm serious I didn't know if something happened to you..." I started crying.

"Aw baby..."

Now the hormones really kicked in.

"You didn't call or leave a note or a message and I've been trying to call you since 5:30 and you didn't answer the phone. When I got home you weren't home and now..."

"Didn't you see my uniform upstairs?" He said hugging me.

"Not right away. I just now realized you were okay when I came into the kitchen and saw your lunch bag, but before then I was starting to think something bad had happened. I even called your job."

"You called my job?"

"Yeah, but nobody answered. I thought maybe if someone was still there that they could at least tell me what time you'd left. I thought you were in an accident because usually when you work late you always call. You didn't call or answer your phone..."

"Alright, I'm okay. I promise it won't happen again."

"You can't be doing this to a pregnant woman." We laughed.

"I didn't have my phone on me."

"Well that's what we got them for goofy. What good are they if we don't use them?"

"Okay, okay, I won't do it again."

"I need a tissue." I headed to the dining room, where we sat down and finished eating. After promising not to mess with the hormonal pregnant lady we had devotions, and then watched TV.

> *"Let them sacrifice the sacrifices of thanksgiving, and declare His works with rejoicing."*
> **Psalm 107:22**

Well tomorrow I will officially be seven months pregnant! I am so excited about this new life, yet I am ever reminded of its fragility. I try not to be afraid and to trust God, but I find this apprehension creeping in. I attended two funerals this weekend, both of young people, and each one reminded me that tomorrow is not promised to any of us.

It didn't help that I also read a true story of a couple who'd lost two babies before successfully carrying one to term. The first one miscarried at five months. She was in severe pain and her water had broken, yet her doctor told her she'd only urinated. Even when her placenta was coming out, he told her it was hemorrhoids and to push them back in. What a tragedy!

She changed doctors for her second pregnancy and this doctor discovered that her incompetent cervix was caused by an unnecessary procedure she'd received years earlier at the hands of her previous Ob-Gyn. Her second baby died in the eighth month from the same thing.
A third agonizing pregnancy came before she successfully carried to term. Her tale was heart wrenching and I could identify with her pain and fears.

What makes me think that I am exempt from this type of suffering? Wanting a child and not being able to have one is one kind of pain, but what about knowing the happiness of carrying a child, only to lose it in the end? Could I handle that?

In my studies on the history of infertility from colonial times until now, I encountered even more tragic stories and of strong men and women who learned to cope. One woman bore twelve children and lost nine of them before they turned a year old. Other women gave up their life savings to charlatan doctors who doled out false hope. Still others endured primitive treatments based more on man's imaginative speculations than actual science.

There were Christian women who like me had to endure the public accusations of *"church women"* levied against them through misinterpretations of God's word that they were somehow cursed because they did not have children. These women were also left to ponder, *"God, what did I do wrong?"* I can't count the number of times I argued with God about it. What more was I supposed to do?"

What makes me any better than them? What makes me think I am immune from more suffering?"

We were watching the news last night and there was a story about millions of people starving in Africa, there were warehouses full of donated food. The news reporter insinuated that the government officials were evil because they would not allow the food to be distributed to the people. Officials believed that it was tainted because it had been chemically altered.

Since no studies existed on the long-term effects, they refused to distribute it, nor would they to allow its seed to be planted on their soil. Daddy said he didn't blame them because once the chemically altered food is introduced into an environment, it takes over completely.

Eventually eliminating all the original forms of it and can destroy the natural ecosystems.

What if the African government were me, and the people *my* children? What would I do if someone gave me something that on the surface seemed good for them, but might actually turn out to be bad?

"Or what man is there of you whom if his son asks bread will he give him a stone? Or if he asks a fish will he give him a serpent? ...
Matthew 7:9-12

Suddenly, I understood. Those leaders were caught in a Catch-22, the precarious position of choosing between the welfare of the current generation, and the destiny of future ones. It wasn't fair. And as usual it all leads back to you.

Why were they born if they were destined to die? What great things will they accomplish? What makes me any surer of my child's future than their parents are of theirs? Why do my children get the privilege of being born a U.S. citizen? What will become of those babies?

My only hope and only comfort, is a blind trust that God did not bring me this far to leave me. I have been fortunate enough to live in a time when medically something could be done about my infertility, but even that would not have been enough had God not stepped in and made a way financially as well.

> *"Bless our children with power and wealth, may they be merciful to those in need, feed the hungry, clothe the naked, and help alleviate human suffering with compassion. May they appreciate what You give them remembering that despite this country's ills; they are still among the worlds most privileged."*

Love Mommy

> *"The Lord is my strength and my shield;*
> *my heart trusts in Him, and I am helped."*
> **Psalm 28:7**

September 9, 2002

Dear Baby Girl:

"You need to start walking if you are going to be in shape for the delivery." Dr. Watson scolded. "You gained ten pounds since your visit last month."

"After all the months of weight loss I'm shocked!" I exclaimed.

"All in all you're not doing too badly; I just want you to be in shape. Delivering a baby is hard work."

"Everybody's gone during the day. I don't have anybody to walk with."

"You'd better go to the mall and walk there." He teased. "You'd better go somewhere."

"How about water aerobics," I asked.

"Water aerobics is good, maybe even better. You just need to start doing something."

"Alright."

"So, you are having a girl." He smiled, "My daughter wants a baby sister so if you don't want her I'll take her."

"I don't think so!"

"Let's check out her heartbeat." He started moving the instrument all over and I was getting nervous watching him and hearing nothing.

"There it is. She's laying traverse, crosswise that is, that's why I was having trouble finding it. Hopefully she will move back into the birth position before your due date, otherwise I will have to perform a C-section."

"Oh, no!"

"We'll see. The important thing is that she comes out healthy."

The weekend of the doctor's visit we went to childbirth education class.

It was a good bonding experience for us. Your daddy enjoyed the breathing exercises because you really moved around a lot during them. The instructor said that the extra oxygen gives babies a rush. Your dad's going to be a good coach and a great daddy.

He boasts, "She'll be one of the few women who'll know how to tune up a car, change the oil, and re-build the engine."

Janet called and asked me how the classes went. "After watching the birth videos I decided that she has to stay in there. But since I know that's not possible I will be taking the epidural. Watching those women who labored and delivered without it I thought, 'What am I crazy?' Obviously there are pros and cons to both, and much respect to the women who go through it without pain medication, but I am not the one." We laughed.

Love Mommy

*"Let us therefore come boldly to the throne of grace
that we may obtain mercy and find grace to help in time of need."*
Hebrews 4:16

September 15, 2002

Dear Baby Girl:

I forgot to tell you the other day I stopped by Jimmy and Staci's to pick up baby pictures of me from mom's old photo albums. I wound up going with them to see Kayla's volleyball game.

At the game you started moving and I let James feel it. I think it sort of freaked him out, because he snatched his hand away and looked away.
"Well he is a little boy that could be kind of freaky." Your daddy said later while working on the house.
"I guess it would be." I said, "So what's on your agenda?" I asked switching gears.
"I'm going to finish stripping the stairs and beating some holes."
"It's illegal to go around stripping and beating 'ho's."
"Lena, that is so corny!" he said, while strapping on his tool belt."
"You're looking pretty sexy in those jeans, T-shirt, and tool belt."
"You can't have me, so don't ask."
"Yeah right, like you'd turn me down if I was!"

I cleaned the house while he stripped the floors. Later, we went to the Mall to pick up the border and curtains for your room. I'm so excited! In general I spent most of the day running errands and by the time I got home I had to pee REALLY, REALLY bad, and that's when it happened! I felt a gush of warm wetness between my legs.

I immediately returned to the rest room to check it out. It didn't look like urine and it looked too watery to be normal vaginal fluid.
"Relax Lena." I said to myself. I went downstairs and calmly said

to your daddy, "Don't be surprised if you have to take me to the hospital."

"Why?" I explained, and then I called the doctor.

Before I could finish talking your daddy had closed all the windows and put away his tools.

"What are you doing?"

"I know you, and no matter what the doctor says you are going to go to the hospital."

"Well, for your information Mr. Smarty man, the nurse told me to go just to be on the safe side. She said it didn't sound as if my water had broken, but since it was still early they'd better check it out."

"Lord, please don't let this baby come now," your dad prayed." we are not ready."

"I know we still don't have the crib."

"That and I don't want her to come so early that we have to leave the hospital without her."

"Oh yeah I didn't think about that."

I kept praying for you to move and you never did. Not during the car ride, registration, or when I went to the restroom to give the urine sample. But when they put that fetal monitor on you went so crazy that even your daddy marveled at the strength of your kicks. It's like you were trying to kick it off. Anyhow, I was just glad to see you moving. See you soon.

Love Mommy

CHAPTER 8

Living Life Without the Secret Shame

*Hope deferred makes the heart sick,
but when the desire comes, it is a tree of life."*
Proverbs 13:12

December 7, 2002

Dear Children:

On Monday, November 18 we went to the doctor praying you'd turned back into the birth position and you did. After my morning appointment Dr. Watson sent me to the hospital, planning to induce labor. When we reached the maternity ward, a very friendly woman introduced us to our nurse who, managed to get us the room we wanted with the adjacent family room. She then hooked me up to all the monitors.

Your aunt Tracee, uncle Craig, and aunt Chrystal took turns coming in to talk to me, while your daddy took pictures and videotaped. After I got hooked up, I had to keep going to the restroom. I kept trying to take off the oxygen mask, but the nurse kept busting me.

Nearly 45 minutes later she still hadn't given me the medicine to induce labor. Every now and then she would come in with the trainee who was shadowing her and look at the results of the fetal monitor. Your daddy got concerned, though it never dawned on me that anything could be wrong.

"Dr. Watson's going to come in himself and give you the medicine," She eventually said. He arrived about 2 PM, looked at the readings.

"Sorry Lena, You're going to have to have a C-section."

"Oh no," I groaned. "Why?"

"The readings from the fetal heart monitor are showing some abnormalities. The nurse noticed them and called me to verify what she was seeing. Every time you have a naturally occurring contraction, the baby's heart rate slows down, putting her in distress. If she can't handle these mild contractions there is no way she will be able to tolerate labor."

"What might cause that?" Your dad asked.

"It could be because she's had a bowel movement in the womb, she has a prolapsed cord (coming first) and it's cutting off her oxygen, or it could mean that her cord is wrapped around her neck. There's no way to know for sure until after the surgery. I do know without the surgery she might not survive the stress of a vaginal delivery."

"Whenever I am afraid I will trust in You."
Psalm 56:3

From there everything happened so fast I hardly had time to think about what was going on.

"So, who's going in with her?" The nurse asked.

"How many people can come?" Daddy asked.

"Three," She said. "But you need to decide quickly."

The next thing I know your daddy, Chrystal, and Mrs. Arnold were being handed scrubs, paper shoes and hats.

"You guys are so slow." I told them.

"I know we've got so much to do to get you prepped." The nurse said.

"No. I am talking about how slow they are getting dressed. You guys are moving fast."

Before they could finish getting dressed, the nurses whisked me to the surgery unit and started the spinal. They tried to move me from the bed to this skinny metal table.

"I need you to try your best and get up to the table and sit on the side.

Do you think you can do it by your-self?" The female anesthesiologist asked.

"Yes, I think so." It still didn't really hit me what was happening. I just focused on the mechanics of the situation.

"Great!" She praised after I got up there. "Now I need you to bend over as far as you can. Try to remain calm." Then she walked me through what was going to happen, while the chief anesthesiologist prepared to perform the actual procedure."

"You're going to have a spinal block." She said, while he prepared the medication. "Do you understand what that is?"

"Yes, but why a spinal and not an epidural," I asked.

"A spinal works faster. Typically an epidural takes 20 minutes to kick in, while a spinal takes only five, and we need to move fast."

I still didn't understand the severity of the situation.

"The doctor is going to give you a local anesthetic to numb the area where the spinal will be administered. This will consist of several pinpricks around the area. It shouldn't feel too bad. After that, the doctor will administer the anesthesia and you shouldn't feel anything."

"I feel so exposed." I said nervously.

"I gave an epidural to my cousin," he said humorously. "She was nervous about me seeing her "*goods,* so to speak, but I assured her that from up here it all looks the same."

"Am I supposed to feel that?" He proceeded to administer the anesthetic.

"Yes, that pressure you feel is completely normal. You are doing so well. You are being so still. That's so great!"

"You mean people actually move during this process?"

"You'd be surprised. Some people are so nervous it's hard to keep them still, I mean they really freak out."

"I'm not about to move anywhere." I remember when mom had to have one when she had cancer. If mom could do it, so could I. She'd gone through much worse, and never complained. I didn't complain either, but the truth is I was terrified!

I lay down and before I knew it I couldn't feel my legs. By then, the three of them entered the room looking calm, but feeling tense.

The anesthesiologist draped a curtain around my midsection, but I could see everything in the big medical lights above me, though I had sense enough not to look.

After they cleaned and shaved me the anesthesiologist started to test for feeling. "Do you feel cold here?" He asked regarding the various places he was rubbing. I don't know what he was using to make me feel the cold, or which of my responses of "yes, no, etc." was the correct marker for determining numbness; I just trusted that he did. He lowered my head, so my legs were elevated; and the medicine would quickly work its way to my abdominal area.

"How are you doing?" Dr. Watson asked, striding calmly and confidently into the room.

"Okay, I guess." Though I hid my anxiety, for fear that if I didn't stay calm I would make something bad happen.

I heard Chrystal and Mrs. Arnold talking to me, but I don't remember what they said. I was there, but it was like I was having an out of body experience or something.

From time to time, your daddy would come over and stroke my head, and I'd hear him say, "*wow*," or something to that effect. He might tell me what they were doing, or tell me how well I was doing.

"I'm getting dizzy, nervous and nauseous. Is this normal?"

"Yes," he said, while asking for something for me to throw up in. He elevated my head and that helped. Your daddy stroked my head, and that helped calm me.

"Do you want to sit down?" I heard your daddy ask his mom.

"What color are your eyes?" The anesthesiologist asked.

"Hazel." I wonder if this a trick question to see if I am coherent.

"Are they real?"

"Yes." I'm too out of it to be insulted.

"They are beautiful!"

"Thank you." I'm too gone to be flattered.

"Can you feel any thing?"

"Not right now but I do have a low pain threshold so I may need more drugs."

"A lady went to the dentist. Just before he came at her with a big syringe, she grabs him between the legs and looks at him, smiles sweetly and says, 'Now we are not going to hurt each other are we?' That's why I'm standing way back here." He says. We all laughed.

"I can't feel my legs."

"You can't feel your legs? Are you seeing a doctor about that?" More laughs. Smiling, he finishes assembling drapes and while he's doing that I could hear Dr. Watson preparing for the surgery.

"You are going to feel a lot of pressure and pulling, but you should not feel any pain. If you do, let me know immediately."

"How are you doing Lena?" Doctor Watson asked.

"I can't feel my legs."

"I told her she ought to see a doctor about that." The anesthesiologist smiled, and I smiled back as best I could.

"I feel shaky." I said uncertainly. There is a lot of chatter as they are preparing.

"It's normal although we really don't know why it happens, perhaps it's a nervous release, but it's normal." He calmly replies. "Just like the tingling and nausea you were feeling earlier."

I was really starting to get terrified. I just lay there trying to stay calm, hoping I would fall asleep, but it did not happen. I could hear everyone talking, but I was just trying not to be there. Before I even knew it I was being cut open and I must have had so much anesthesia that I barely felt the tugging and pulling I'd been warned I'd feel.

"Where does he think he's going?" I said watching the anesthesiologist leave the room.

Then I heard the doctors conversing about everything but me, just like they do on those doctor shows. "I'm like could you focus please, after all I am lying here all cut up!" I guess they are so good that they can do that. They're talking about the hospital, their practices, their family, music, golf, the Flintstones, etc.

They worked fast! Within minutes of being cut open you were out and I could hear you crying. It wasn't really until that moment that it all became real to me.

I mean I knew you were in there, but until I actually heard you cry all I could think about was death. Even after I heard you wail it was hard to focus on the joy. The experience was nothing like I thought it would be.

None of the videos warned me about all the mental crap I'd go through. In the videos, the mothers were given their babies right away, even after a C-Section. In my real world, I didn't even get to see you until after they cleaned you off, and then it was only for a few seconds.

I'd like to tell you that I cried just like those mothers in those videos, but I was out of it. I even didn't get to hold you until an hour later.

"Are you sure you are my child?" I said looking at you.

"She's going to start hollering in a minute, and then you'll know she's yours." Your dad joked.

"What are you trying to say?" I asked weakly.

"Well, that big old head is all yours."

"I can't believe how big she already is. Look at those hands and feet!" Chrystal exclaimed.

"Eight pounds, seven ounces, she is a big baby, but, hey she got it honest, she's got a big mamma. But she's beautiful!"

"Look at her licking her lips like she wants a pork chop." Mrs. Arnold said.

"Try to feed her." Chrystal said.

"I don't think I have the energy to put her there, but I'll try." That and I didn't want to whip my booby's out in front of them. Nevertheless I tried, and to your credit so did you, but neither one if us could hang.

Everybody and their mama showed up in that recovery area until the nurse finally ran some of them off. Then the pediatric nurses whisked you away for your first full check up. I was still waiting for feeling to return in my legs; terrified the entire time that it wouldn't come back. I never really thought about how a paraplegic feels until that moment.

I wondered how I was going to take care of my baby if my legs didn't come back. I told you, you think of all kinds of crazy stuff.

After about an hour your dad and grandma came back from the nursery.

"How did she do?" I asked.

"She was quiet at first, but then she got to yelling up a storm when bath time came. They are going to bring her to the room later."

"Alrighty then, I can't wait!"

"Well Lena, now that you've had a baby, what are you gong to do?" Janet asked later that evening.

"We'll as much as I'd love to; I'm not going to Disney World."

"Does it seem real yet?"

"It's been a wild ride; my emotions ran the gamut from extreme happiness to utter fear and confusion."

"All of that is normal. I've been there."

Around 11 PM your daddy and I finally got to be alone with you and I sang my little song to you while your daddy taped.

"So how does it feel to finally be a mommy?"

"Aside from the fact that I can't feel my legs and I'm in pain-It feels GREAT! I think she has your nose and she snores like you. God I can't believe all this came out of me!" I said staring at you. "It's so weird; the whole process of childbirth still amazes me. I mean the fact that another human being can carry another one inside them and deliver this whole other person. Think about it. Where does the tissue come from, bones, hair, muscle, etc.? I mean I know the science of it, but even science can't really explain it all. It's just God!"

"It's amazing! So, what are we gonna name her?"

"You want Éva, then Éva it shall be."

"Well. I've got another woman in my life." He said, while we fell asleep on him.

Love Mommy

"...You formed me in my inward parts"
(Psalm 139: 13-18)

Thursday, November 21

Dear `Eva:

"HeyLenawhat'sgoing on?Howareyoufeeling?I'msohappyforyou!" Felecia said in one breath. "Are you feeling okay?"

"I'm just battling fatigue. The pain wasn't too bad because they kept me on a pain pump the first night. They removed the IV line today, but they bring me pills regularly to keep the pain at bay. It's really uncomfortable when I have to move, walk; go to the restroom or shower, which they make me do as much as I can. I didn't do much today though."

"You had a C-Section right? How did it go for you?"

"I hated it!"

"Really? I loved mine. The only thing I didn't like was having that catheter."

"That wasn't too bad. The C-Section was rough. I know it had to be done; it's just that I wasn't psychologically prepared for the ordeal. I should have been because you always know it's a possibility, but when she turned I threw the idea out of my head, you know?"

"It does make a difference." She said. "I knew going in I was going to have one, so I had plenty of time to prepare mentally."

"I mean, I read about things, and watched videos, and they all prepare you for the mechanics of the procedure, but none truly prepare you for the roller coaster of emotions and feelings you go through. It was the most stressful situation I have ever been in. I felt totally overwhelmed and out of control."

"Really, wow I didn't feel that way at all, but like I said I did have time to prepare. Maybe I would've been the same way if it had come on suddenly like yours."

"Yeah, I mean I went in thinking I was going to deliver natural and the next thing I know I'm being whisked away to an operating room. I was scared-no *terrified*, and at one point during the operation I felt like I couldn't catch my breath."

"Did you tell them that?"

"No, I didn't say anything because I was afraid I'd make my heart rate drop. That sounds crazy doesn't it? I told my doctor later and he said my breathing was fine. He said, 'It was worth it wasn't it? You have a healthy, beautiful baby girl who looks just like her daddy.' It worked out though 'cause as big as she was I don't know if my vagina could've handled it!"

"Other than that, how are you feeling?" She asked laughing.

"Except for the occasional loss of dignity things are pretty cool, so far. Like when I was in the shower and one of the nurses walked right in to give me some medicine like it wasn't anything. I'm like, "I'm standing here buck naked okay!" Let's not even talk about the enema administration. I'm turned over on my side in pain, while two strangers probe my private parts, oh, the humanity!"

"Oh yeah girl I remember that! At first I was like, people please, I'm in here naked, can I have some privacy? I guess they have seen it all, but it's still new to you. After a while I just didn't care who saw what."

"I know. The only downside here is the nurses."

"Why?" Felecia asked.

"Some of them make me think the baby is going to die if I don't breastfeed her every hour. All she wants to do is sleep and they try to force me to wake her up."

"Oh yeah, I had similar issues."

"It's like there is a war going on in this hospital."

"Let me guess, some say, "Let her alone and let her sleep."

"Yep. I call them the *Breast Rebels.*"

"Then the others tell you, 'Oh, you've got to wake her every three hours to eat. No you cannot supplement with formula or a bottle, you don't want to cause nipple confusion.'"

"Those are the *Titty Patriots.*"

"Girl that is funny."

The *Titty Patriots* wouldn't bring me a breast pump and the *Breast Rebels* secretly fed you at night. Well la de da, thanks for telling me I mean I am only her mother. I'm her mother! Omigosh, I am a mother!

A worried mother!

"She has some slight jaundice," the pediatrician said. "I'll have them run some tests tomorrow morning to check the levels and make sure she's okay. Other than that she's fine."

"What about all the puffiness and drainage from her eyes. They look like they are infected?" I asked.

"There's nothing wrong with them," he said. "Some puffiness and drainage is normal at birth, but if it doesn't clear up, we'll check it again."

"Why is her skin so dry?"

"She's okay, but get some lotion from the nurses, because they won't put any on if you don't ask."

Hearing about the jaundice almost brought me down, but he assured me you were fine. My good time went downhill from there.

By the time Dr. Watson arrived I wanted to ask for a sedative.

"Hi Lena, how are you doing?" He smiled. "I've been in surgery; otherwise I'd have been here a while ago."

"It's no problem with me." I smiled as best I could.

"Are you feeling okay?" He asked as he motioned for me to lie down so he could check my incision.

"I don't know. I'm starting to feel nauseous, I have a headache, and my feet are still swollen. I'm a little concerned about all that."

"That's all normal, I assure you." He said. "Good news you can go home and take care of that pretty baby."

"Thanks again for everything. I know I'm a hypochondriac and sometimes I give you a hard time, but I really appreciate all you have done for us."

"You're welcome, and you're not a hypochondriac, just a new mother. Now take a deep breath and relax. It will be all right. You have a beautiful baby."

"Okay."

"I want you to call the office and schedule an appointment for two weeks from today, okay."

Shortly after Dr. Watson left, already feeling scared and unsure, Chrystal called to ask what was going on.

"Dr. Watson just finished examining me and I'm officially discharged. Horace is on his way to pick me up."

"What did the pediatrician say about her jaundice?"

"The doctor personally called and said she was fine. He said that the levels were in the acceptable range and that this was normal for a newborn. He said it usually clears up in a couple of days, but to keep an eye on her. As long as she's eating well, she'll be okay. I accepted that and thanked him. She has a doctor's visit on Tuesday and he's going to check on her again then, but he said not to worry unless she stops eating."

"What does *an acceptable range* mean?"

"I don't know, I guess it means it's okay since that's what he said."

"You need to find out."

"Well the nurse just walked in, I'll ask her to check 'Eva's chart and let me know what the range was."

"I was on the Internet reading about jaundice and depending on what her levels were it could range from moderate to severe; with severe meaning she could die, so you need to find out." She said giving me all the worst-case scenarios.

Okay, I'm already not feeling well, I'm worried about her eating, the Titty Patriots are driving me crazy, and now this! I couldn't take it anymore! I just started crying.

"I'm sorry I didn't mean to upset you." She said pretty freaked out by my sudden outburst. "Calm down, Marie it's going to be okay."

"It's not just that I am simply experiencing information and well-meaning advice overload. I'm already growing anxious about being a mother and all these people are giving me all this conflicting advice and I didn't know what to do, and I miss my mother…"

"Okay Marie calm down okay…"

"The nurse is here to check on me and finish discharging me; I'll have to call you back when I get home."

I stood over the bassinet looking at you. By now I was feeling totally overwhelmed and out of control. I just stood there looking at you on the verge of bursting into more tears.

"Are you alright?" I heard the nurse ask.

"No," I said bursting into more tears.

"What's wrong?"

I tried to explain without sounding like an incoherent idiot. Somehow, through all the sniffling and tears she understood and comforted me.

"They all mean well," she said kindly.

"And while there is a measure of truth in all they say, you are this child's mother and you should do what you think is best for her. Okay."

"Okay." I sniffed, unable to say more. You would have thought I was fifteen instead of thirty-something. "On top of all the stress I think I'm just missing my mother." I said as she worked. "I never thought she wouldn't be here when I had kids, you know?"

"Did your mom die of cancer?"

"Yes, how did you guess that?"

I don't know. My mom died of cancer several months ago, so I totally understand. She was there for me when I had my children, but I don't know what I would have done if I had to go through childbirth without her. I'd probably be the same way." By the time she left the room, we were both crying.

The first day of your homecoming I was still in a fog, but by the second day I was crying out to God to help me deal with the overwhelming emotions that threatened to cripple me. Yeah, that's right, Post Partum Blues kicked in.

"This poor man cried, and the Lord heard him, and saved him out of all his troubles."
Psalm 34:6

There were times I felt like I was going to pass out as my hormones readjusted. Hot flashes, night sweats, and anxiety attacks, all seemed to hit at once. No one but Sharon and Janet, who'd gone through it too, knew how overwhelmed I was. I desperately missed my mother and I cried constantly.

I didn't know what to do with you. I cried some more. You cried to the point of choking and I freaked out and handed you to daddy.

Then I cried because I panicked and because I am your mother and I felt I should have been able to calm you and I couldn't.

Then I tried not to cry because I was afraid doing so would make me feel worse and heighten the sense of anxiety and fear. So I prayed because that's all I knew how to do. Then I called Janet, who made me give the phone to your daddy. She told him to keep an eye on me and if I didn't get better in a day or so, call the doctor and get me some medicine.

"The LORD bless you and keep you; The LORD make His face to shine upon you, and be gracious to you; The LORD lift up His countenance upon you, and give you peace."
Numbers 6:24-26

Then she told me. "Lena, there is nothing wrong with praying and I know God can bring you through, but there is nothing wrong with taking the medicine either. Normal Post Partum resolves itself within a few days. If you are not back to yourself within that time frame-get some help!" She wouldn't let me hang up until I promised to do so.

I thank God for my friends, and I thank God that Jesus is my friend, because having Jesus means that I will always have someone who:

> *loves me unconditionally.*
> *sticks by me.*
> *understands me.*
> *holds me accountable.*
> *surrounds me with wisdom*
> *comforts me.*
> *sees beyond my faults.*
> *will never forsake me.*
> *thinks about me.*
> *shares secrets with me.*
> *will keep all my secrets.*

I took her advice and allowed myself the time I needed to grieve for my mom and air my concerns to God. He held me in His arms and soothed my pain. Thankfully it resolved itself within the three day time frame.

Then I prayed for your well being. That nothing would happen to you until we knew that you would be okay without us.

I looked down into your bassinet and hesitantly picked you up and held you. And in that moment I felt God, and knew that holding you close was like holding my mom. I then felt the peace of God. I would have taken the medicine if I needed it because I know Post Partum Blues can be serious, but thankfully the anxiety abated, and I could finally enjoy the thing I had been praying for-which was you!

Love Mommy

The Finish

When your dreams have been broken in pieces
and your hopes appear as glass shattered
Remember, it's not how you started,
it's how you finish that matters.

Though through the course of this life you may falter
and the end seems nowhere in sight
Remember, the sun always arises,
to displace the dark of the night.

Through faith there are mountains to conquer
and yes valleys yet to go through.
Yet if we but trust in the Master
no dream is too lofty for our hearts to pursue.

Hope is contained in the spirit
that believes on broken wings it can still fly.
Towards the new life in tomorrow,
as it tosses today's torments aside.

In this life as we strive for perfection
some dreams may become broken and shattered.
But Remember, it's not how you started,
it's how you finish that matters.

Lena Arnold

Epilogue

My Christian experience might be different than most as I was baptized as a Catholic, raised in Pentecostal Holiness, gave my life to Christ in a Baptist church, studied eastern and western religions in college, and served for ten years in what now would be considered an Evangelical environment.

However, there is one truth that remains steadfast among them all. They all believe that God is omnipotent, and that he possesses the power to heal. The debates begin when discussing how he chooses to use that power, particularly in the area of assisted reproductive technology.

One belief system scorned the very idea, making the thought synonymous with serving the devil. Still another taught that if you just prayed hard enough, everything would work itself out. One had no answers, but allowed no room for the questions.

Because I didn't have a sickness the leaders could identify with and the answer to my illness seemed to cross the boundaries of ethical religious practices. And that stifled us for a long time.

The day came when we had to seek God for ourselves. At our disposal was the Bible, our personal relationship with God, scientific knowledge, and my friend's husband who was both a Christian and a physician.

Utilizing all the resources in our arsenal we concluded that it was God who gives man knowledge and the power to use that knowledge for good or evil. We understood our desire to procreate was in fact very Biblical, and therefore we were well within our rights to seek the help that many religious leaders had scorned.

According to the Centers for Disease Control and Prevention, more than 9 million women have used infertility services, and over 6.1

million people of reproductive age in this country are infertile.

The National Center for Health Statistics approximates that of 4.5 million couples who experience infertility yearly only 2 million actually seek help.

There are many causes of infertility and it is recommended that couples, in which the female partner is over age 35, should seek help after 6 months of being unable to conceive. Couples who already have known causes of infertility are advised to seek help even earlier.

On average ordinary couples are advised to talk with their doctor one year after they begin actively attempting to achieve a pregnancy.

Deciding when to seek help is often a difficult decision for couples to make, but I encourage you to follow the recommendations above. **Don't wait like we did**. The sooner you begin the process the sooner you can begin regaining control of your life.

And while you may not be able to control the outcome, you can control how you deal with the process. The sooner you can begin to deal with the process, the sooner you can remove the mask and begin living your life to the fullest.

Then you can go on, trusting that whichever way God turns you will be the direction ordained for you from before the foundation of the world; and in doing so you will regain a sense of power over your malady.

I encourage you to visit my website, **www.*IN*fertilitypress.com** for more information on coping with and overcoming infertility.

Love Lena

About the Author

LENA ARNOLD is a respected consultant on family and youth issues and has spent the last 20 years working tirelessly on their behalf. She is primarily responsible for helping non-profits & businesses achieve organizational goals through the creation of effective development strategies.

As a graduate of the Wright State University School of Liberal Arts, she began her career as a, journalist and has written for several periodicals within the Dayton community where she currently resides. For this Child We Prayed represents her second foray into the world of professional book publishing. The first being a joint effort with InSCRIBEd Inspirations, entitled Free to Fly: Reflections on Womanhood.

Lena is consistently sought out as a motivational speaker for her dynamic public speaking abilities.

For more information, please visit **www.*IN*fertilitypress.com**.

Resources

The Word In Life™ Study Bible: New Kings James Version Published by Thomas Nelson, Copyright 1993, 1996

A Treasury of Wisdom Journal, Compiled by Angela Abraham, Barbour and Company, Inc.

"*The Power of A Praying Parent,*" by Stormie Omartian, *Single Parent Family Magazine*, August 1996

Elizabeth L. Marshall, "*Conquering Infertility*," Franklin Watts Library

Sandra Glahn and Dr. William Cutrer, "*When Empty Arms Become A Heavy Burden: Encouragement for Couples Facing Infertility*," Broadman & Holman Publishers, 1997.

Margaret Marsh & Wanda Ronner, "*The Empty Cradle: Infertility in America From Colonial Times to the Present,*" John Hopkins University Press, 1996

Arlene Eisenberg, Heidi Murkoff & Sandee Hathaway, B.S.N., "*What to Expect When You're Expecting,*" Workman Publishing

Glade B. Curtis, M.D., OB/GYN & Judith Schuler, M.S., "*Your Pregnancy After 35,*" Perseus Publishing, 2001

Mary Lou Ballweg and the Endometriosis Association, "*The Endometriosis Sourcebook,*" Contemporary Books, 1995

The Warrior Is A Child, from the CD entitled *A Heart That Knows You* by Twila Paris © *Copyright,* 1995 Star Song Communications

Why from 4HIM's Face the Nation CD, © *Copyright* 1998, Verity

No Way, No Way (You Won't Lose) from Fred Hammond and Radical for Christ, *Pages of Life* CD © *Copyright* 1998, Verity Face To Face

"*Living in the Land of AND,*" sermon by Dr. Marva L. Mitchell, Pastor Revival Center Ministries International, Copyright 1996 (*used by permission*)

Informative Notes

Page 23
Per Dr. Mark Bidwell, Parlodel is not stronger than Clomid. It treats a different problem that may affect fertility-a high prolactin level. Prolactin is a hormone from the pituitary gland that normally controls breast milk production-may be elevated when it is not supposed to be. There is no "stronger" fertility pill than Clomid. The next stronger thing is an injection of gonadotropins.

Page 107
Progesterone levels are checked one week after IUI to measure quality of ovulation. A pregnancy test is performed two weeks after the IUI if no period has come.

Page 124
Sperm washing is a 2 hour process preparing the sperm for fertilization by carefully removing dead sperm and debris.

Websites

Depression After Delivery Inc. : www.postpartum.net

Postpartum Support International: www.behavenet.com

RESOLVE: www.resolve.org

International Council for Infertility Information Dissemination (INCIID): www.inciid.org

Directory of the American Society of Reproductive Medicine: www.asrm.org

The Endometriosis Organization: www.endo-online.org

U.S. Department of Health and Human Services
Centers for Disease Control and Prevention
National Center for Health Statistics
www.aapps.nccd.cdc.gov/art99/nation99.asp

The American College of Obstetricians and Gynecologist: www.acog.com

Women's Surgery Group: www.womenssurgerygroup.com

A Special Thank You To:

InSCRIBEd Inspiration
"Helping writers find their creative voice."

InSCRIBEd Inspiration Offers:

- ➢ Editing Services
- ➢ Business Development
- ➢ Publishing Services

For more information contact:
Penda James, Editor/Publisher
InSCRIBEd Inspiration
Pittsburgh, PA
(412) 362-6223

Unique Wellness Resource Center
Helping Families and Individuals Maintain Optimum Health
6601 N. Main Street
Dayton, OH 45415
(937) 559-9155

Notes & Comments

www.ingramcontent.com/pod-product-compliance
Lightning Source LLC
Chambersburg PA
CBHW051432290426
44109CB00016B/1523